Integrated View of Population Genetics

Edited by Rafael Trindade Maia and Magnólia de Araújo Campos

Published in London, United Kingdom

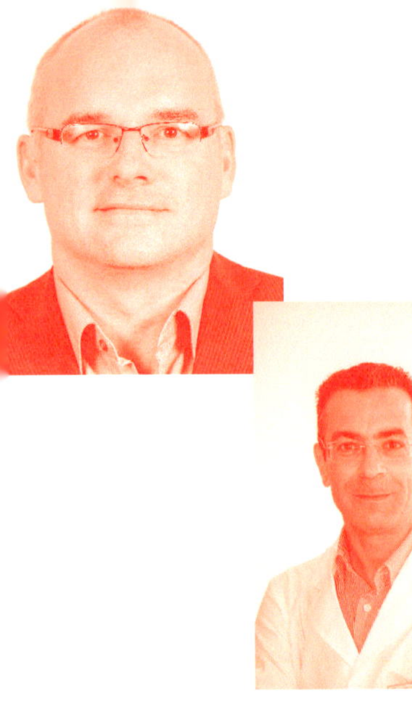
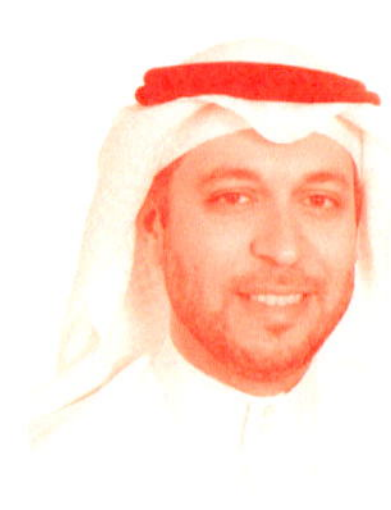
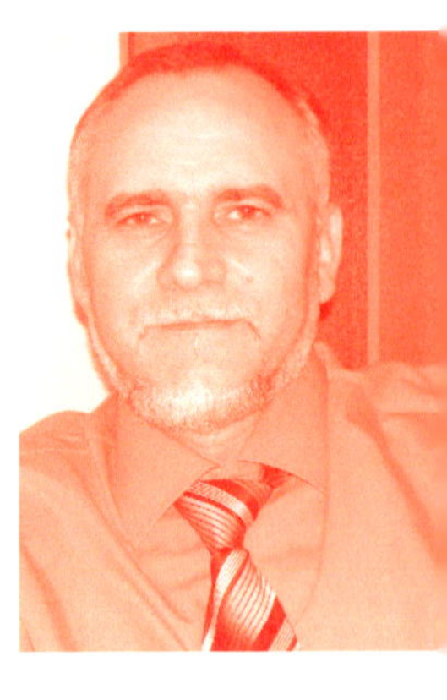
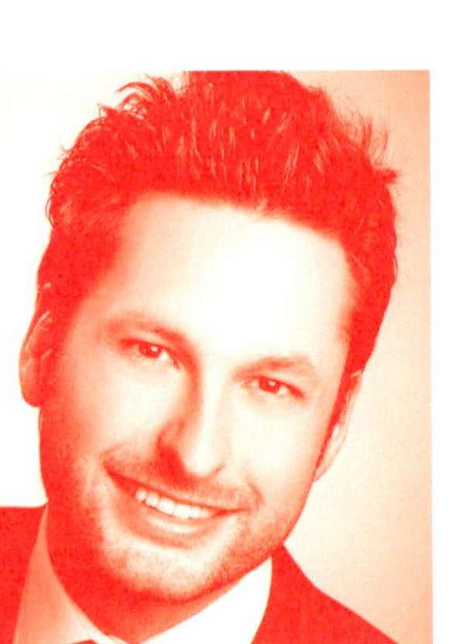
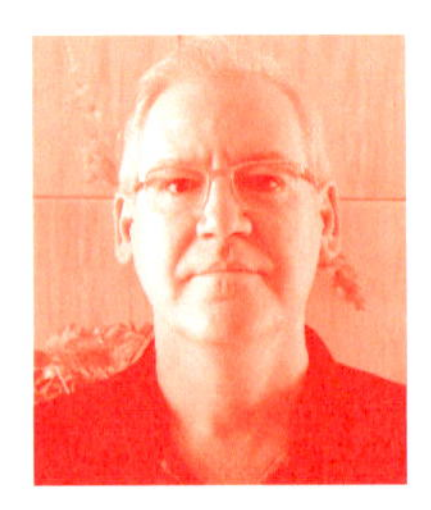
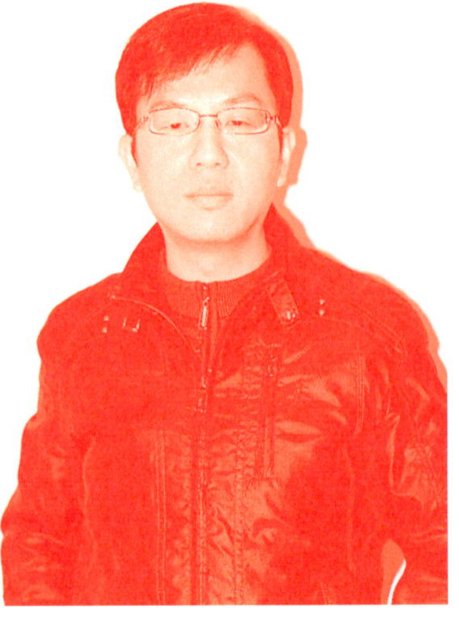

IntechOpen

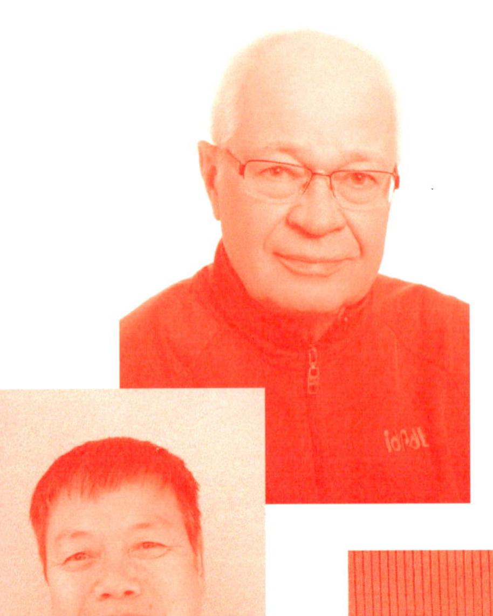
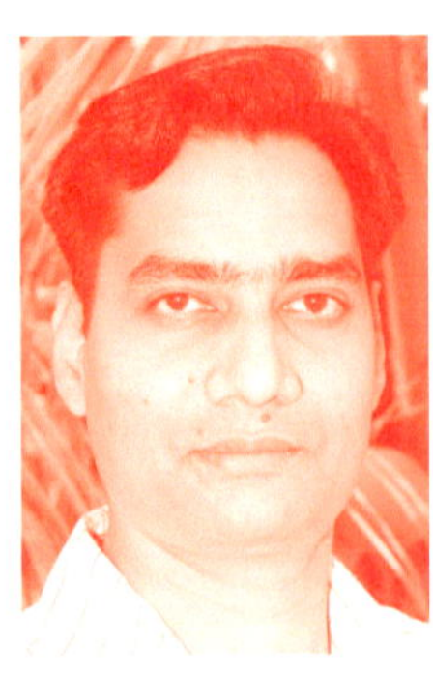
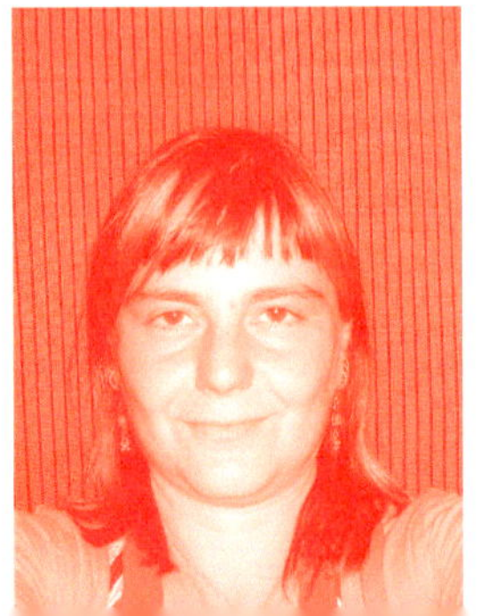
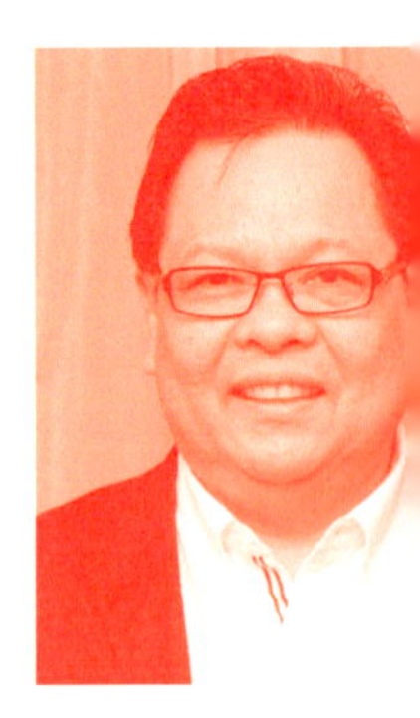
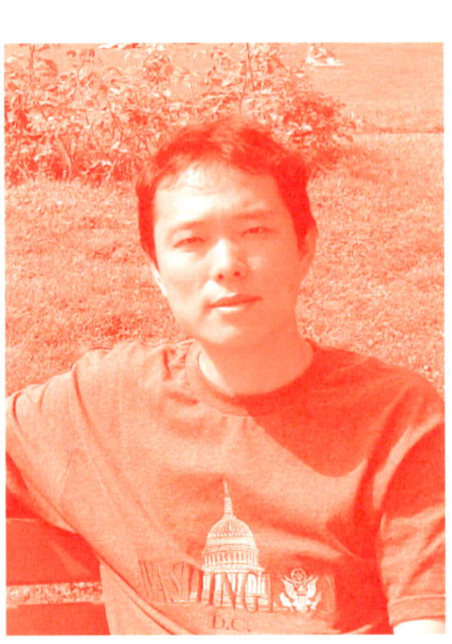

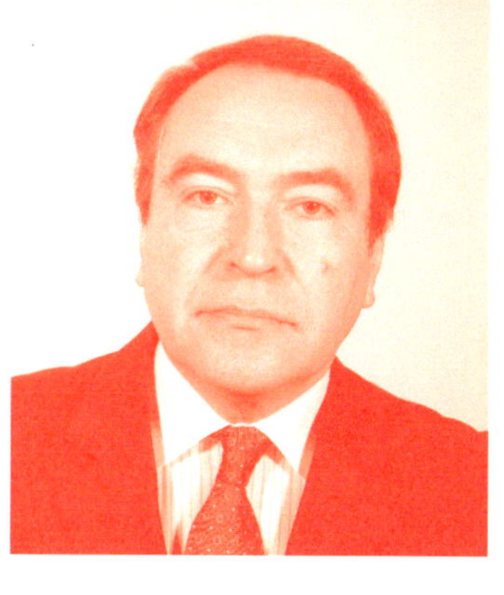
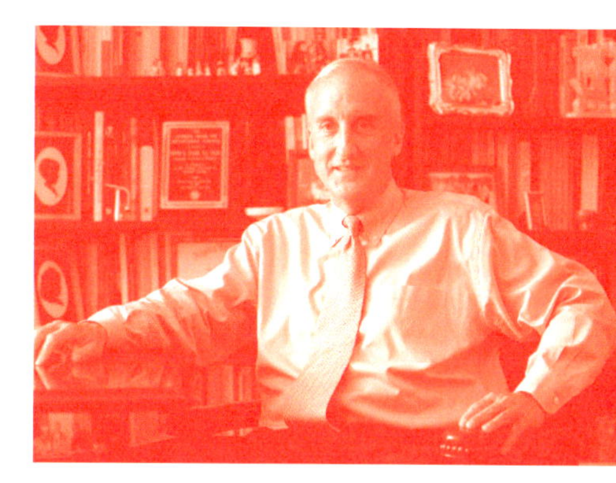
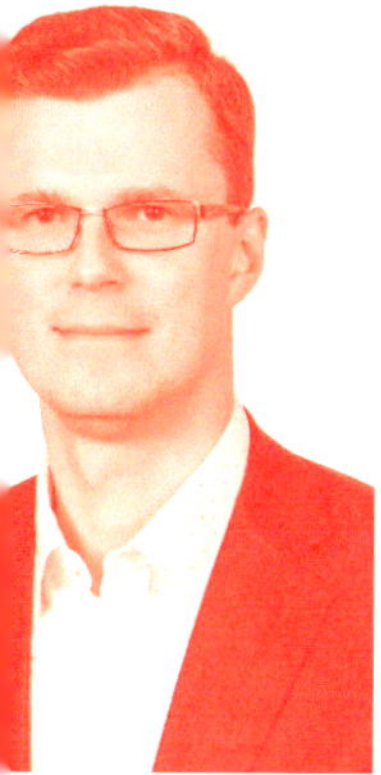
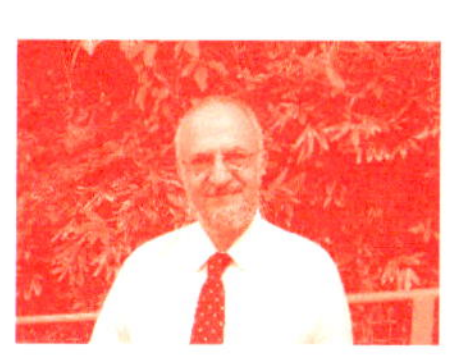
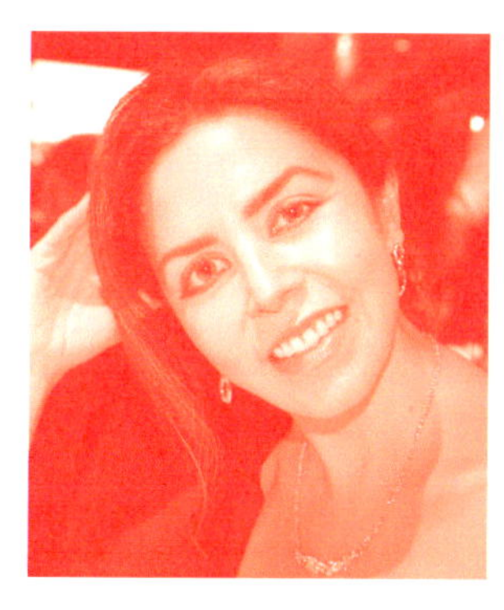

Supporting open minds since 2005

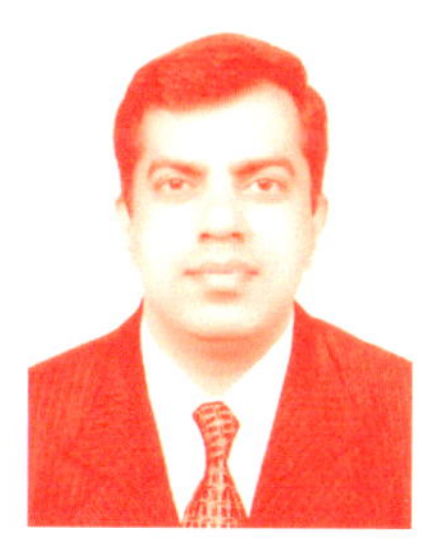
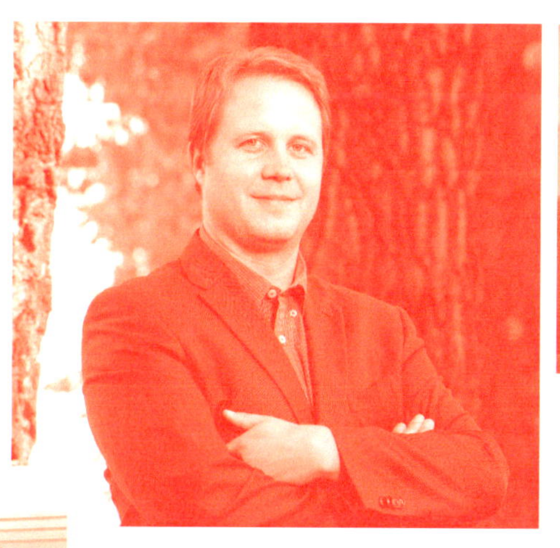
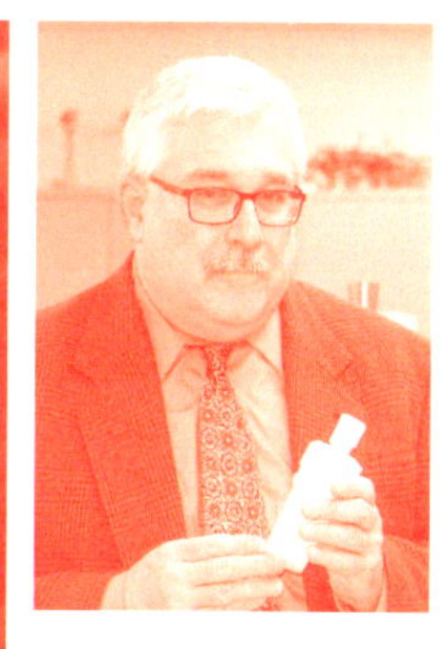
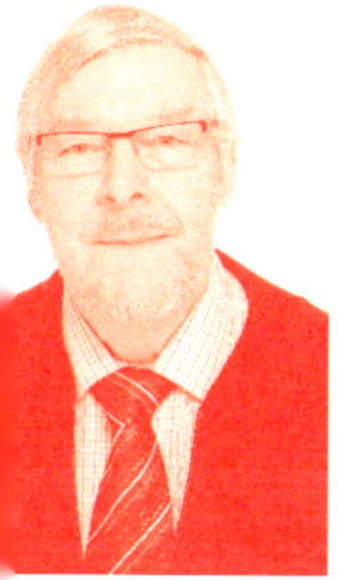
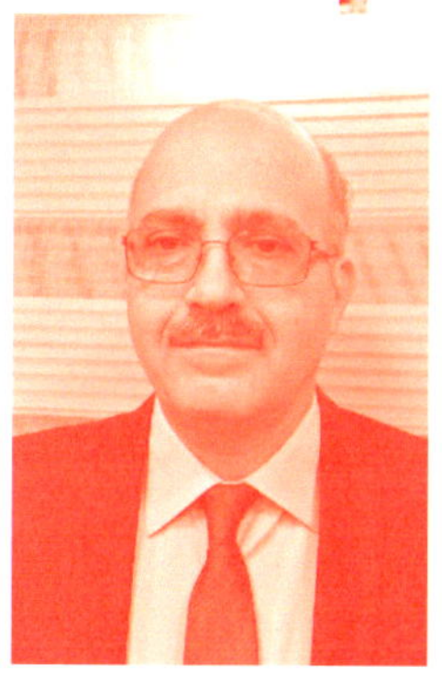
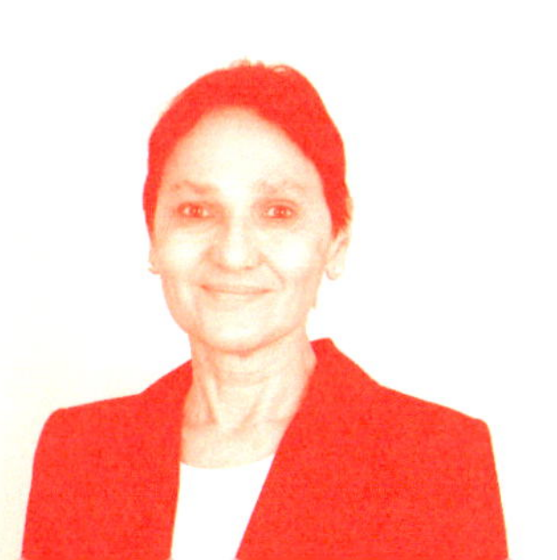
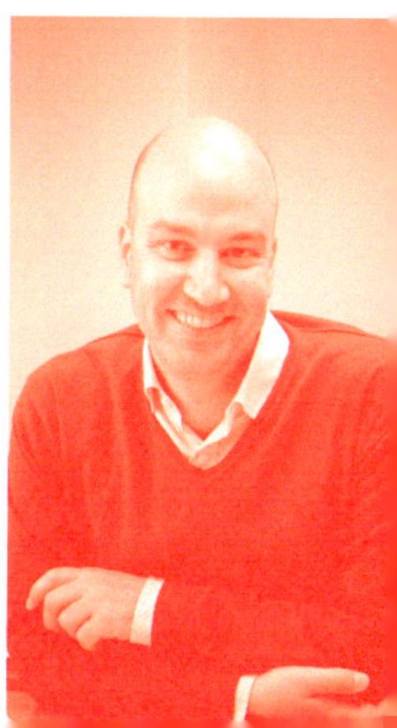

Integrated View of Population Genetics
http://dx.doi.org/10.5772/intechopen.73721
Edited by Rafael Trindade Maia and Magnólia de Araújo Campos

Contributors
Inés Hugalde, Cecilia Aguero, Sebastián Gomez Talquenca, Hernán Vila, Summaira Riaz, Andrew Walker, Yongshuang Xiao, Zhizhong Xiao, Jing Liu, Daoyuan Ma, Qinghua Liu, Jun Li, Te-Ming Tseng, Swati Shrestha, Shandrea Stallworth, Rafael Trindade Maia

First published in London, United Kingdom, 2019 by IntechOpen
IntechOpen is the global imprint of INTECHOPEN LIMITED, registered in England and Wales, registration number: 11086078, The Shard, 25th floor, 32 London Bridge Street
London, SE19SG - United Kingdom
Printed in Croatia

British Library Cataloguing-in-Publication Data
A catalogue record for this book is available from the British Library

Additional hard copies can be obtained from orders@intechopen.com

Integrated View of Population Genetics
Edited by Rafael Trindade Maia and Magnólia de Araújo Campos
p. cm.
Print ISBN 978-1-78985-777-1
Online ISBN 978-1-78985-778-8

For EU product safety concerns:
IN TECH d.o.o., Prolaz Marije Krucifikse Kozulić 3, 51000 Rijeka, Croatia, info@intechopen.com or visit our website at intechopen.com.

Meet the editors

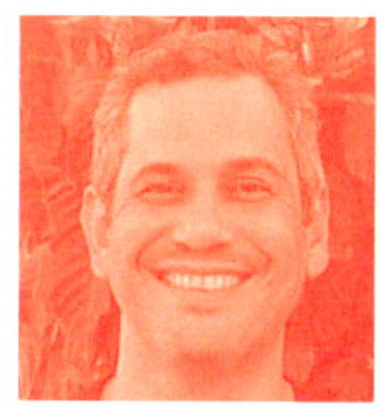

Rafael Trindade Maia graduated in with a Bachelor's degree in Biological Sciences from the Federal Rural University of Pernambuco (2005), a Master's degree in Genetics, Conservation and Evolutionary Biology from the National Research Institute of the Amazon (2008), and a PhD in Animal Biology from the Federal University of Pernambuco (2013). He is currently a professor at the Center for the Sustainable Development of the Semi-Arid (CDSA) of the Federal University of Campina Grande (UFCG). He has experience in population genetics, bioinformatics, molecular docking, modeling, and molecular dynamics of proteins. He works in the area of science and biology education. He leads the research groups Computational and Theoretical Biology (BCT) and Teaching of Sciences and Biology (ECB).

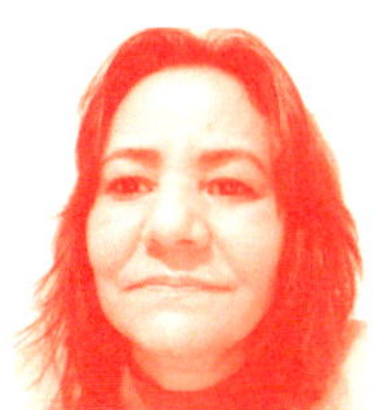

Magnólia de Araújo Campos graduated with her Bachelor's degree in Biological Sciences from the State University of Paraíba, a Master's degree in Agronomy/Phytomedication from the Federal University of Pelotas, and a PhD in Biological Sciences/Molecular Biology from the University of Brasília. She is an Adjunct Professor at the Federal University of Campina Grande (UFCG), and currently develops activities at the Center for Education and Health (CES, Campus Cuité). She is a coordinator of the Academic Master's Course in Natural Sciences and Biotechnology at the CES/UFCG. She has experience in vegetable tissue culture, plant transgenics, molecular markers, bioinformatics, genomics, in vitro heterologous expression of antimicrobial proteins, and plant and molecular biology of microorganisms. She is currently working on projects involving the following themes: host-pest molecular interaction, proteins related to defense, genetic prospecting, and secretoma.

Contents

Preface

Population genetics is a fascinating branch of biology that focuses on the analysis of distribution and changes in the allelic frequencies of populations. Since its inception as a science in 1966, population genetics has advanced significantly due to the development of new molecular techniques, mathematical-statistical models, new software, and genomic databases. Currently, several theoretical and applied studies use the innumerable tools of population genetics for various inferences, analyzing the genetic structure of organisms for a better understanding of the dynamics of their populations.

This relatively recent science has important applications for the management of populations (natural and domesticated) as well as for evolutionary studies of the various factors that affect gene frequencies over time and across the world.

This book presents relevant results from carefully selected and evaluated population genetics studies and is presented in the form of chapters.

In the first chapter, the editors make a brief and objective presentation on population genetics, with an emphasis on the evolutionary processes that cause changes in the allelic and genotype frequencies in populations.

The second chapter deals with a study of the mapping of vigor genes in wine grapes as a quantitative (polygenic) inheritance, characteristics associated with the storage capacity of carbohydrates, and also the high metabolism and rapid development of these plants.

In the third chapter, the authors present a review addressing a series of genetic factors associated with the characteristics of interest for breeding one of the world's most important cultivars, rice.

The fourth chapter is about a study with AFLP markers applied to studies of populations of a fish species of commercial interest, with implications for adequate management of fish stocks, actions that aim to minimize inbreeding, and decrease of genetic diversity in these populations.

Rafael Trindade Maia
Federal University of Campina Grande, Sumé-PB, Cuité, PB, Brazil

Magnólia de Araújo Campos
Federal University of Campina Grande, Sumé-PB, Cuité, PB, Brazil

Section 1

Introduction

Chapter 1

Introductory Chapter: Population Genetics - The Evolution Process as a Genetic Function

Rafael Trindade Maia and Magnólia de Araújo Campos

1. Introduction

Population genetics is defined as the sub-area of biology that studies the distribution and change in frequency of alleles. The population genetics is also the basis of evolution, and it has been established as a science; its main founders were JBS Haldane, Sir Ronald Fisher, and Sewall Wright. Since 1966, from the pioneering work of Fisher, Haldane, and Wright, the population genetics had accumulated a large mathematical theory, statistical tools, laboratory techniques, molecular markers, and huge information of polymorphisms in databanks [1]. The main concept in population genetics is focused on the Hardy-Weinberg theorem (also known as Hardy-Weinberg theorem or Hardy-Weinberg law). This central theorem preconizes that if the population size is large, with random mating, and mutation, selection, and migration are not significant, the allelic frequencies do not change over the generations. If not, the allelic and genotype frequencies will change from one generation to the next. These changes can affect directly in population's adaptive fitness, so information for applied studies and decisions can be provided by accessing the genetic variation in populations.

2. Evolutionary processes that interfere on genepool

Population genetics is an extremely useful tool for studies of microevolution, population dynamics, and conservation genetics. When accessing the genetic constitution of a population, several parameters can be conserved such as phenotypic frequencies, genotype frequencies, allelic frequencies, gene flow, heritability, genetic correlation, genetic diversity, heterozygosity, and several other indicators that allow an understanding of the genetic dynamics of the population in study. Through this information, it is possible to improve strategies for proper management and control or even more efficient conservation actions.

Among the evolutionary processes that interfere in the gene pool of populations, altering their genetic constituent, they include mutation, migration (with gene flow), natural selection, and genetic drift [2].

Mutation is the classic source of genetic variation, generating new alleles in a population. They direct the evolution and have different probabilities depending on the type of mutation, and this has implications for the evolution of genotypes. For example, if a G-A mutation occurs more frequently than A-G genotypes with the nucleotide A tend to be more common in the population. In summary, one can classify the mutations at synonymous and non-synonymous, that is, those that

IntechOpen

entail changes in amino acid and those which do not cause changes in the peptide chain, also called neutral mutations. According to the theory proposed by Kimura neutrality, most mutations which attach the populations are of neutral type, since most non-synonymous mutations cause deleterious effects on the phenotypes of individuals [3].

Genetic drift is the change in gene frequency due to an event of random selection of individuals, usually in small populations (**Figure 1**). Genetic drift can have serious consequences for the population and can cause alleles to permanently disappear from a population, reducing their genetic variability. Drift can occur in two ways: the founder effect and bottleneck effect. The founder effect is the decrease of genetic diversity due to a new population established by few individuals [4, 5],

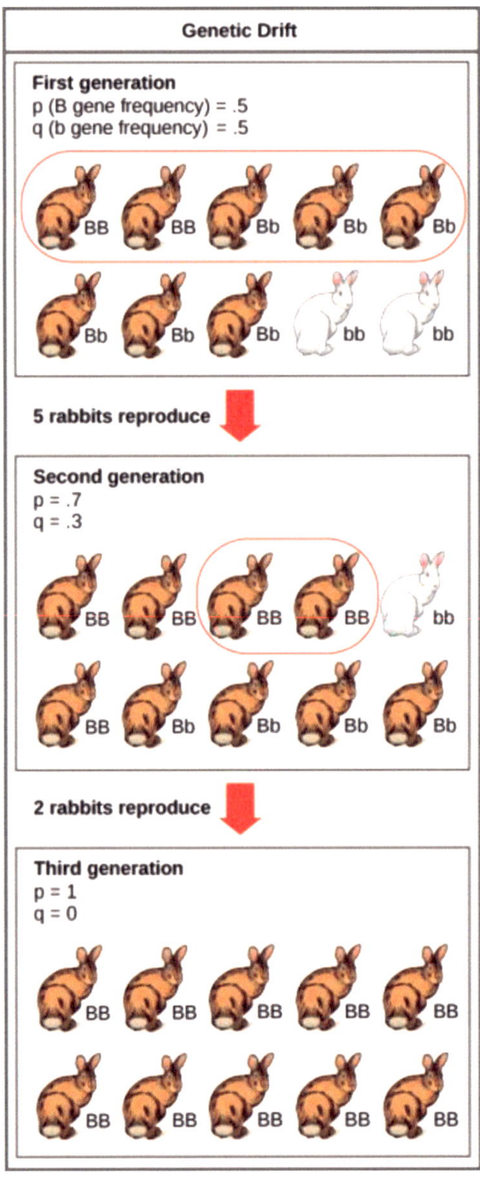

Figure 1.
Genetic drift. Source: Google images.

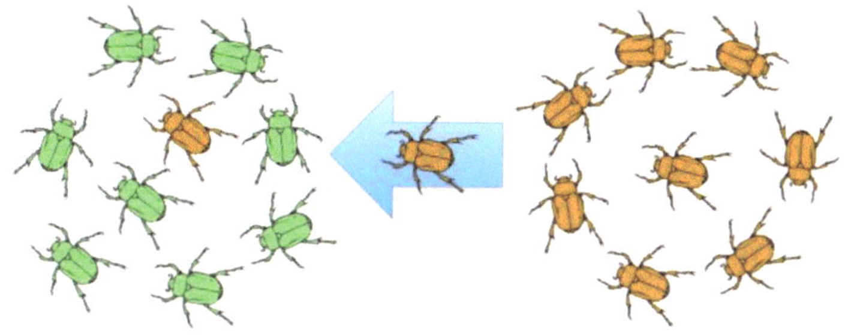

Figure 2.
Migração com fluxo gênico. Source: Google images.

while bottleneck effect is the reduction of population size by environmental events (earthquakes, famines, floods, disease, fires, or droughts) [6].

The impacts of genetic drift in a population will vary according to the effective population size (N_e), which can be estimated by the following equation:

$$N_e = \frac{4 N_f N_m}{N_f + N_m} \tag{1}$$

where N_e is the effective population, N_m is the number of breeding males, and Nf is the number of breeding females.

Migration with reproductive success (**Figure 2**) allows the introduction of new alleles into the population, thus altering their genetic structure. Gene flow is one of the main parameters to evaluate the degree of structuring between populations of the same species [7].

Natural selection, a process observed by Charles Darwin, is the adaptation of organisms to the environment. It acts through the selection of genotypic changes in a given population. Through natural selection, mutations that increase the chances of individuals surviving and procreating tend to be preserved and multiplied in populations (positive selection), and mutations that decrease population fitness (deleterious mutations) tend to be eliminated (purified selection).

The future of population genetics is very promising. The crucial progress in this field has showed that today, it is particularly relevant for the comprehension of genetic variation among populations from many species. Advances in population genetics will impact strongly the way we deal with biodiversity, pathogenic species, crops, and many other species.

Author details

Rafael Trindade Maia* and Magnólia de Araújo Campos
Universidade Federal de campina Grande, Sumé-PB, Cuité, PB, Brazil

*Address all correspondence to: rafael.rafatrin@gmail.com

References

[1] Charolesworth B, Charles Worth D. Population genetics from 1966 to 2016. Heredity. 2017;**118**:s2-s9

[2] Kimura M. The Neutral Theory of Molecular Evolution. Cambridge: Cambridge University Press; 1983

[3] Gillespie JH. Population Genetics. A Concise Guide. Baltimore/London: The Johns Hopkins University Press; 1998. pp. 19-48. 169 páginas. ISBN: 0-8018-5755-4

[4] Provine WB. Ernst Mayr: Genetics and speciation. Genetics. 2004;**167**(3):1041-1046

[5] Templeton AR. The theory of speciation via the founder principle. Genetics. 1980;**94**(4):1011-1038

[6] William RC Jr. Bottleneck: Humanity's Impending Impasse. USA: Xlibris Corporation; 2009. pp. 290. ISBN: 978-1-4415-2241-2

[7] Frankham R, Briscoe DA, Ballou JD. Introduction to Conservation Genetics. Cambrige: Cambridge University Press; 2002. ISBN: 9780521639859

Section 2

Population and Quantitative Genetics

Chapter 2

Studying Growth and Vigor as Quantitative Traits in Grapevine Populations

Inés Pilar Hugalde, Summaira Riaz, Cecilia B. Agüero, Hernán Vila, Sebastián Gomez Talquenca and M. Andrew Walker

Abstract

Vigor is considered as a propensity to assimilate, store, and/or use nonstructural carbohydrates for producing large canopies, and it is associated with high metabolism and fast growth. Growth involves cell expansion and cell division. Cell division depends on hormonal and metabolic processes. Cell expansion occurs because cell walls are extensible, meaning they deform under the action of tensile forces, generally caused by turgor. There is increasing interest in understanding the genetic basis of vigor and biomass production. It is well established that growth and vigor are quantitative traits and their genetic architecture consists of a big number of genes with small individual effects. The search for groups of genes with small individual effects, which control a specific quantitative trait, is performed by QTL analysis and genetic mapping. Today, several linkage maps are available, like "Syrah" × "grenache," "Riesling" × "Cabernet Sauvignon," and "Ramsey" × *Vitis riparia*. This last progeny segregates for vigor and constituted an interesting tool for our genetic studies on growth.

Keywords: PCA, QTL mapping, vegetative vigor, biomass partitioning, quantitative trait

1. Introduction

In 1865, Mendelian studies gave birth to genetics as a science. The Mendelian model accurately explains inheritance for qualitative traits, with discontinuous distributions. But, what happens with quantitative, continuous traits, like growth or vigor? These quantitative, polygenic, complex traits reveal the expression of many genes with small but additive effects. The part of the chromosome where these genes are clustered is called quantitative trait loci or QTLs.

The main economic interesting traits, like production, growth, and vigor, have quantitative distributions and respond to QTLs. In addition, as they are being controlled by many genes, similar phenotypes may have different allelic variations, or plants with the same QTLs may have very different phenotypes in different environments. Additionally, the epistatic effect, caused by allelic combinations of different genes—meaning that the expression of a certain gene may affect the expression of another—adds variations in the final expression of the phenotype.

Sax [1] was the first to describe the theory of QTL mapping. Later, Thoday [2] suggested that it was possible to apply the well-known concept of segregation of simple genes, to linked QTL detection. The vital participation of molecular markers that have been developed through the years allowed improving the technique, permitting, in many cases, the identification of a certain gene or few genes responsible for the quantitative phenotypic variation [3]. In a very elegant thesis, Donoso Contreras [4] adopts the "needle in the hay" analogy to picture the difficulty in finding, in a whole genome, one gene with quantitative effect. QTL analysis allows dividing the hay into several "bunches of hay" and systematically looking for the "needle."

QTL analysis links two types of information—phenotypic data (measurements) and genetic data (molecular markers)—in an attempt to explain the genetic bases of variations in complex traits [5, 6]. This analysis allows linking certain complex phenotypes to certain regions in the chromosomes. The original premise is to discover locus by co-segregation of the phenotypes with the markers.

Two things are essential for QTL mapping. In the first place, two contrasting parents for a certain trait are crossed, and a segregating population must be obtained. Later, genetic markers that distinguish the two parental lines are involved in the mapping. In this sense, molecular markers are preferred as they will rarely affect the studied trait. The markers linked to a QTL that influences the character or trait of interest will segregate with the trait (in high-frequency, lower recombination rate), while the non-linked markers will segregate separately (high recombination). For highly heterocygous species, like grapevines, to obtain pure homocygous lines is almost impossible, and the F1 progenies that do segregate are feasible to be studied. This progenies are called pseudo F1 progenies.

There are three statistic methodologies for the detection of a QTL: single marker analysis, simple interval mapping (SIM), and composite interval mapping (CIM). In the first case, single marker analysis, the technique is based on ANOVA and simple linear regression. It is simple and easy to do, not needing a genetic map as it analyzes the relation between each marker with the phenotype. On the other hand, SIM uses a genetic map to define the interval among adjacent pairs of linked markers [7]. Finally, CIM is combined with SIM for a single QTL in a given interval with multiple regression analysis of associated markers to other QTLs, including additional genetic markers or cofactors that control the genetic background. This is the most efficient and effective approach [8]. The results of QTL analysis are presented in terms of logarithm of the odds (LOD) scores or probabilities [9]. Strictly, a QTL is considered significant when its LOD score is higher than the LOD score calculated by permutation tests [10]. After localizing the QTL, the explained variability is calculated by means of the average values of the phenotypes of the genetic groups of the QTL, in the position of the map with maximum LOD score [3].

1.1 Vigor as a quantitative trait

Vigor is considered the genotype's propensity to assimilate, store, and/or use nonstructural carbohydrates for producing large canopies, and it is associated with intense metabolism and fast shoot growth [11, 12]. Carbon assimilation (A) turns to be the vital mechanism that makes growth possible. For A to occur, CO_2 must diffuse into the leaf mesophyll, through opened stomata. The trade-off of C assimilation is loss of water from the leaf to the atmosphere. This inevitable water loss through opened stomata (and the depreciable diffusion through cuticle) constitutes transpiration (E). This means that A and stomatal conductance (g_s) are tightly correlated [13] and stomata are directly responsible for optimizing E *vs.* A [14].

Growth involves cell expansion and cell division [15]. Cell expansion takes place when cell walls deform under the action of tensile forces, generally caused by turgor

DOI: http://dx.doi.org/10.5772/intechopen.82537

[16]. The plant water uptake capacity is influenced by the hydraulic conductance (k_H) of the roots which in turn confers different hydration and turgor to the canopy [17, 18], conferring different growth levels by cellular extension [19]. Keller [20] found that k_H adapts to support canopy growth and carbon partitioning but may limit shoot vigor in grapevines. These differences in k_H that account for variation in growth among genotypes have a genetic correlate. Marguerit et al. [21] detected quantitative trait loci (QTL) for E, soil water extraction capacity, and water use efficiency (WUE) when studying water stress response of *Vitis vinifera* cv. Cabernet Sauvignon × *Vitis riparia* cv. Gloire de Montpellier progeny. They observed that their QTLs co-localized with genes involved in the expression of hydraulic regulation and aquaporin activity that directly affect the plant k_H, as previously proposed [18].

There is increasing interest in deepening on the genetic basis of vigor and biomass production. It is well stablished that growth and vigor are quantitative traits and their genetic architecture consists of multiple genes with small individual effects. Today, several linkage maps are available, like Syrah × grenache, Cabernet Sauvignon × Riesling, and Ramsey × *Vitis riparia* [22–24]. Lowe and Walker concluded that the Ramsey × *V. riparia* linkage map was a valuable tool with which to examine and map traits like biotic resistance, drought tolerance, and vigor. This map was used to study vigor and map QTLs in relation to this trait.

2. Physiological component of vigor

In 1997, under code 9715, in the University of California, Davis, a cross between Ramsey (*Vitis champinii*) and *Vitis riparia* Gloire de Montpellier (**Figure 1**) was done. The purpose of this cross was to study biotic resistances. Later, it was observed that the population also segregated for vigor and vegetative growth, among other quantitative traits [24]. This allowed the opportunity of inquiring about the genetic and mechanistic bases of this characteristic.

This population is a pseudo F1 cross of Ramsey and *V. riparia* GM. In grapevine, the high heterozygosity makes it impossible to recover pure homocygous lines and obtain F2 crosses or backcrosses. Segregation is possible in pseudo F1 populations. In this way, our F1 from Ramsey and *V. riparia* GM was obtained with the intention of studying biotic and abiotic resistances and vigor.

One hundred thirty-eight genotypes from a F1 progeny between Ramsey and *V. riparia* GM were evaluated at UC Davis, California, in the summer of 2014 and 2015. Shoot growth rate (b); leaf area (LA); leaf, shoot, and root dry biomasses (DWL, DWS, DWR); plant hydraulic conductance (k_H); root hydraulic

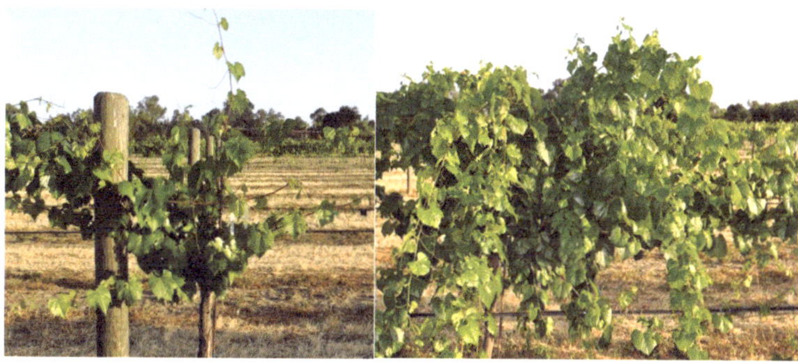

Figure 1.
Two extreme genotypes from the Ramsey (Vitis champinii) and Vitis riparia Gloire de Montpellier. UC Davis, Davis, CA, USA.

conductance (Lp_r); stomatal conductance (g_s); and water potential (Ψ) were measured as vigor-related traits. Specific leaf area (SLA: LA/leaf biomass) was calculated, and QTL mapping and detection were performed on both parental and consensus maps. A complete description of the techniques and methods used to measure and assess the variables studied is published by Hugalde et al. [25].

Hydraulic variables were not mapped, as they were measured in a smaller number of genotypes given the time-consuming nature of the methods that asses them. However, significant statistics evidenced an important role of root hydraulics in vigor definition [25].

A principal component analysis (PCA) of a subset of 50 genotypes explained 80% of the variability (**Figure 2**). Component 1 showed strong positive effects of LA, growth rate (b), and root dry weight (DWR), while strong and negative effect was found for specific root hydraulic conductance (L_{pr}, hydraulic conductance per gram of dry biomass). This negative effect explains that more vigor corresponds to lower L_{pr}, meaning that smaller plants and smaller root systems tend to be, when considered per biomass weight, more effective in water absorption than vigorous plants. This was also observed by Lovisolo et al. [26] in olive dwarfing rootstocks, Herralde et al. [17] when studying grapevine rootstocks under water stress, and Kaldenhoff et al. [27] with *Arabidopsis thaliana* and an antisense construct targeted to the PIP1b aquaporin gene. Later, similar results were observed in kiwi plants, where leaf area-specific conductance and g_s were both higher in the low-vigor rootstocks [28]. Finally, one more study with two chickpea progenies showed the same type of behavior, being the low-vigor plants the ones with higher root hydraulic conductivity and higher transpiration rates [29]. This higher Lp_r in small root systems of low-vigor plants seems to try to compensate the low biomass production, while vigorous plants, which may be less efficient per biomass unit, have bigger root systems, with more biomass accumulation, and in conclusion higher total root hydraulic conductance.

For component 2, positive effects were explained by specific leaf area (SLA) and the partitioning index constituted by leaf area (LA) and total biomass. SLA is an

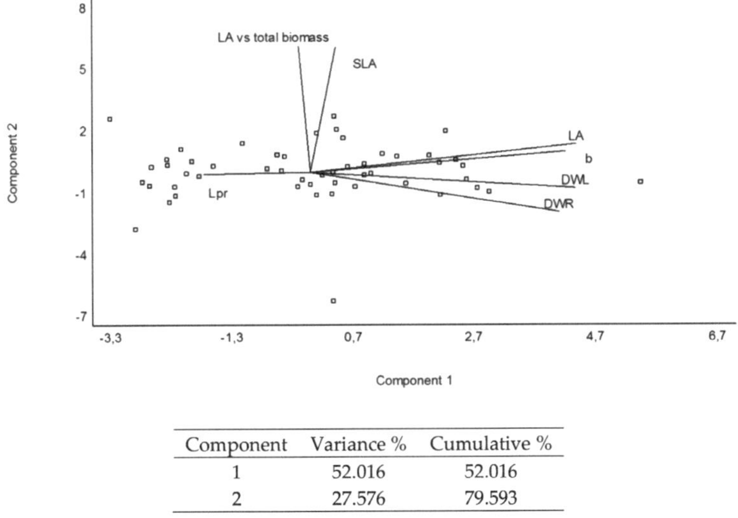

Component	Variance %	Cumulative %
1	52.016	52.016
2	27.576	79.593

Figure 2.
Principal components analysis of the main phenotypic characters related to vigor under well-watered conditions in 2015. L_{pr}, root-specific hydraulic conductance; b, stem growth rate; SLA, specific leaf area; DWL, leaf dry weight; DWR, root dry weight; LA, leaf area; LA vs. total biomass, partitioning index. N = 50 [25]. This analysis was carried out with Statgraphics centurion XVI, 16.1.11.

important parameter of growth rate because the larger the SLA, the larger the area for capturing light per unit of previously captured mass. These indices indicate that different genotypes with different vigor also have different partitioning pathways; as for vigorous plants, more LA *vs.* total biomass can be expected, while for smaller plants, the opposite is expected. However, when comparing dry weights (biomass), low-vigor plants tend to have small canopies and also small root systems. This clearly shows how LA, which depends on leaf biomass and the hydraulic situation (turgor that allows cell expansion), is so different between opposite genotypes. Big plants with higher total plant hydraulic conductance have more leaf area, with respect to their biomasses, than small plants [25].

3. Genetic component of vigor: QTL mapping in a grapevine population

The Ramsey × *V. riparia* GM progeny showed transgressive segregation and significant differences between small, intermediate, and big plants. **Figure 3** shows vigor (canopy biomass, B) for the complete progeny and the parents, for 2014. Data for 2015 (not shown) showed similar results [25].

For *V. riparia* GM, during the first year of study, 16 significant QTLs at the chromosome level were found (LOD scores higher than the threshold value calculated after 1000 permutations, for α 0.05), but only three resulted significant genome wide (LOD scores higher than the threshold calculated for the genome). The partitioning indices related to canopy *vs.* root biomass were significant at the group level and considered putative (**Table 1**).

For LA *vs.* total plant biomass and SLA, QTLs explaining 11.4 and 9% of variance were found in chromosome 1, next to a putative QTL for LA. For LA, another QTL, explaining 12% of total variance, was found in chromosome 4.

During the second year of study and mapping, the parental map of *V. riparia* GM showed five QTLs, significant at the chromosome level (**Table 2**). This time, chromosomes 4 and 16 showed once more QTLs for traits related to biomass partitioning and LA. This result allowed us to have good confidence about these QTLs, previously considered as putative, but found in two independent mapping processes. On the other side, for variables like SLA and growth rate, new QTLs were found during 2015.

For the parental Ramsey map (**Table 3**), during 2014, the first year of mapping, seven putative QTLs were found. LA/total biomass, SLA, and partitioning indices

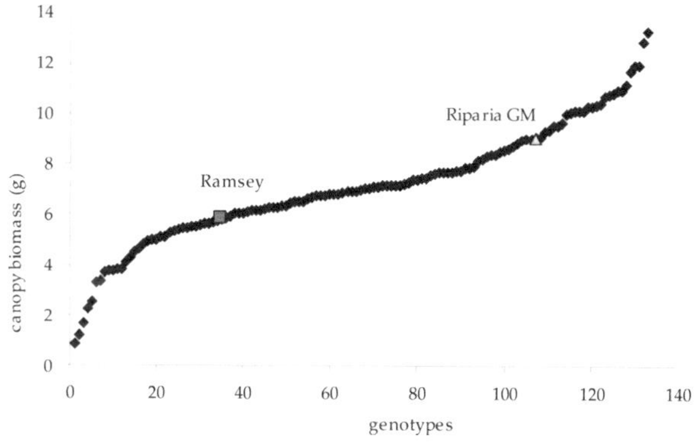

Figure 3.
Vigor (canopy biomass) for the complete progeny and the parents for 2014 [25].

Chromosome	Trait	LOD	Chromosome LOD threshold	Explained variance (%)	Genome LOD threshold
1	**LA/total biomass**	**3.3**	**1.5**	**11.4**	2.6–2.8
	LA/DWR	2.13	1.5	7.5	
	SLA	**2.6**	**1.5**	**9**	
	LA	2.03	1.6	8	
4	**LA**	**3.48**	**1.6**	**12**	
	Total biomass	2.15	1.6	8	
	Canopy	1.93	1.6	7	
	DWL	2.39	1.7	9	
16	DWR/DWS	1.8	1.6	7	
	DWR	1.96	1.6	7	
5	DWR/total biomass	2.45	1.5	8.5	
	Canopy/total biomass	2.45	1.5	8.5	
	DWS/total biomass	2.02	1.5	7	
	Canopy/DWR	2.44	1.5	8.5	
19	Stem growth rate (b)	1.55	1.5	6	

Bold letter indicates genomewide significance for the trait.

Table 1.
QTLs for the V. riparia GM parental map in 2014 [25].

Chromosome	Trait	LOD	Chromosome LOD threshold	Explained variance (%)	Genome LOD threshold
7	LA/total biomass	1.95	1.6	7	
	SLA	2.08	1.6	8	
15	Stem growth rate (b)	2	1.3	7	2.6–2.8
16	DWS/total biomass	1.63	1.3	6	
4	**LA/total biomass**	**2.32**	**1.7**	**9**	

Bold letter shows significant traits for 2014 and 2015, related to LA.

Table 2.
QTLs for parental V. riparia GM map in 2015.

were mapped. No QTLs for LA, growth rate, canopy, or total biomass could be detected.

During the second mapping, in 2015, Ramsey showed 21 QTLs (**Table 4**), among which four were genome-wide significant, being all the rest considered as putative (significant at the chromosome level). Among these putative QTLs, it is worthy to mention that the mapped traits were LA, growth rate, canopy, and total biomass, also found in the Riparia map. In addition, one of the putative QTLs corresponded to shoot biomass (DWS), also found in chromosome 14, in 2014. The four genome-wide significant QTLs were found in chromosomes 1 and 19 of the Ramsey map, corresponding to partitioning variables like DWR/DWL, DWR/total biomass, canopy/total biomass, and LA/total biomass. This last trait, which explains 11% of the phenotypic variance, has almost the same biological meaning as SLA, as it represents the possibility of the plant to transform biomass from its "whole body," into sunlight-receiving screen, for photosynthesis. This variable was mapped in

Chromosome	Trait	LOD	Chromosome LOD threshold	Explained variance (%)	Genome LOD threshold
13	LA/total biomass	2.05	1.4	7.5	2.7–2.8
	LA/DWR	2.28	1.4	8	
	SLA	1.45	1.3	5	
	DWS/total biomass	1.47	1.4	5	
14	DWL/total biomass	2.21	1.9	8	
	DWS/DWL	1.93	1.8	7	
	DWR/DWL	2.05	1.9	7	

QTLs for parental Ramsey map in 2014.

Table 3.
QTLs para el mapa de Ramsey para 2014.

Chromosome	Trait	LOD	Chromosome LOD threshold	Explained variance (%)	Genome LOD threshold
14	DWS	2.23	1.7	8	2.5–2.8
	Canopy	1.83	1.7	7	
	LA	**1.91**	**1.8**	7	
	Number of leaves	2.25	1.8	8	
	Growth rate b	2.25	1.7	9	
9	DWR	2.23	1.5	8	
	Total biomass	1.62	1.4	6	
6	DWR/total biomass	1.6	1.6	6	
	Canopy/total biomass	1.73	1.5	6	
	Canopy/DWR	2.08	1.7	8	
1	Canopy/DWR	2.43	1.6	9	
	DWR/DWS	2.38	1.6	9	
	DWR/DWL	2.68	1.6	10	
	DWR/total biomass	2.86	1.6	10	
	Canopy/total biomass	2.86	1.7	10	
19	SLA	2.05	1.5	8	
	LA/total biomass	**3**	**1.4**	**11**	
8	DWS/DWL	1.52	1.3	5	
17	DWS/DWL	1.52	1.2	5	
4	DWS/total biomass	2.33	1.6	9	
	LA/total biomass	1.89	1.7	7	

Bold letter shows genomewide significant traits and LA related traits.

Table 4.
QTLs for the parental Ramsey map in 2015.

Chromosome	Trait	LOD	Chromosome LOD threshold	Explained variance (%)	Genome LOD threshold
1	LA/total biomass	3.39	2.8	12	4
	SLA	3.23	2.8	11	
13	**LA**	**2.8**	**2.8**	**10**	
4	**LA**	**3.67**	**2.7**	**12.5**	
3	Canopy	2.95	2.5	10	
	DWS/DWL	2.64	2.4	9	
	DWL/total biomass	2.64	2.5	9	
	DWL	3.82	2.5	13	
	Total biomass	3.04	2.5	10.4	
11	**LA**	**2.9**	**2.7**	**10**	
5	DWR/DWL	2.92	2.4	10	
	DWR/total biomass	3.38	2.5	11.5	
	Canopy/total biomass	3.38	2.6	11.5	
	Leaf density	3.41	2.5	12	
10	Canopy/DWR	2.85	2.6	10	
7	Leaf density	3.65	2.7	12.5	

Bold letters show traits related to LA.

Table 5.
QTLs for consensus maps for 2014.

Chromosome	Trait	LOD	Chromosome LOD threshold	Explained variance (%)	Genome LOD threshold
6	DWR	2.83	2.8	10	
3	**LA**	**2.75**	**2.6**	**10**	
1	DWR/DWL	3.16	2.8	11	
	DWR/total biomass	2.82	2.8	10	4.2
	Canopy/total biomass	2.82	2.8	10	
17	DWS/total biomass	2.81	2.6	10	
19	**LA/total biomass**	**4.28**	**2.7**	**15**	

Bold letters show genomewide significant traits.

Table 6.
QTLs for consensus map (2015).

chromosome 19, along with SLA, probably evidencing that it could be possible that the same genes encode for both traits.

Consensus maps of both mappings are shown in **Tables 5** and **6**.

Consensus map from 2014 (**Table 5**) showed significant QTLs at the chromosome level, but not genome wide. There was positive interaction in chromosomes 5 and 7 for leaf density and in chromosomes 5, 4, and 13 for LA, variables that were not mapped in the parents. In these consensus maps, significant QTLs were also mapped

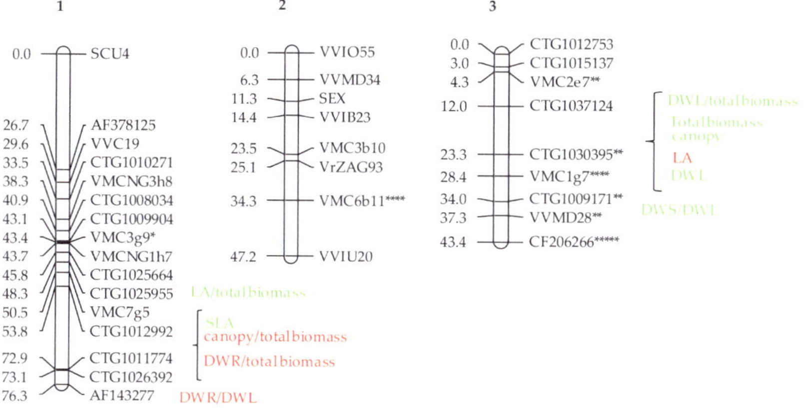

Figure 4.
Consensus linkage map from Ramsey and Riparia Gloire de Montpellier. Chromosomes 1–3. In green, QTLs mapped in 2014. In red, QTLs mapped in 2015.

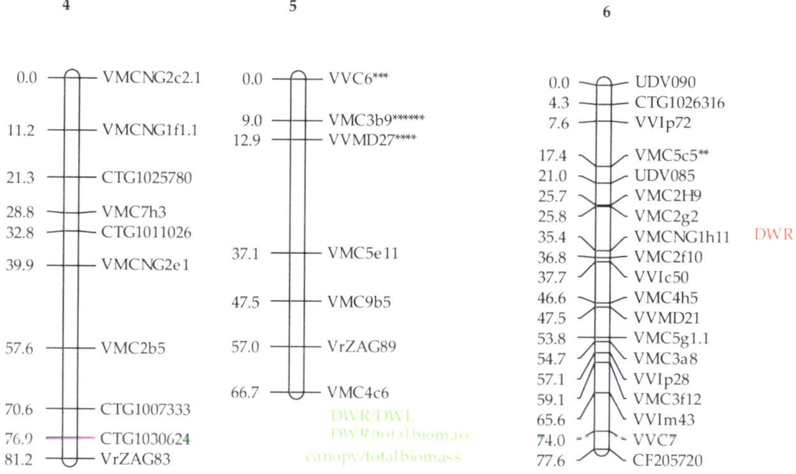

Figure 5.
Consensus linkage map from Ramsey and Riparia Gloire de Montpellier. Chromosomes 4–6. In green, QTLs mapped in 2014. In red, QTLs mapped in 2015.

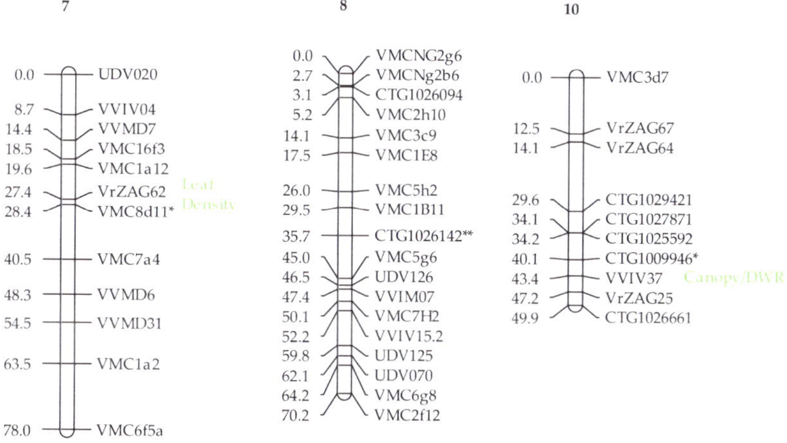

Figure 6.
Consensus linkage map from Ramsey and Riparia Gloire de Montpellier. Chromosomes 7–10. In green, QTLs mapped in 2014.

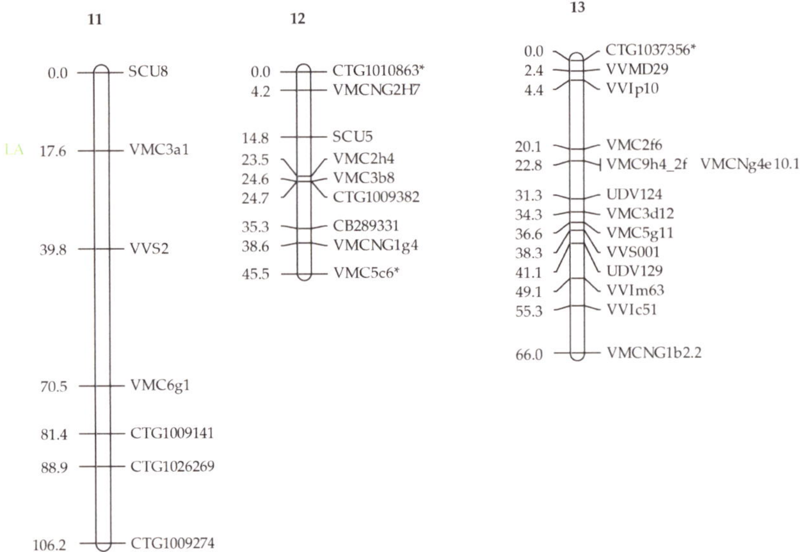

Figure 7.
Consensus linkage map from Ramsey and Riparia Gloire de Montpellier. Chromosomes 11–13. In green, in chromosome 11, QTLs mapped in 2014 for LA.

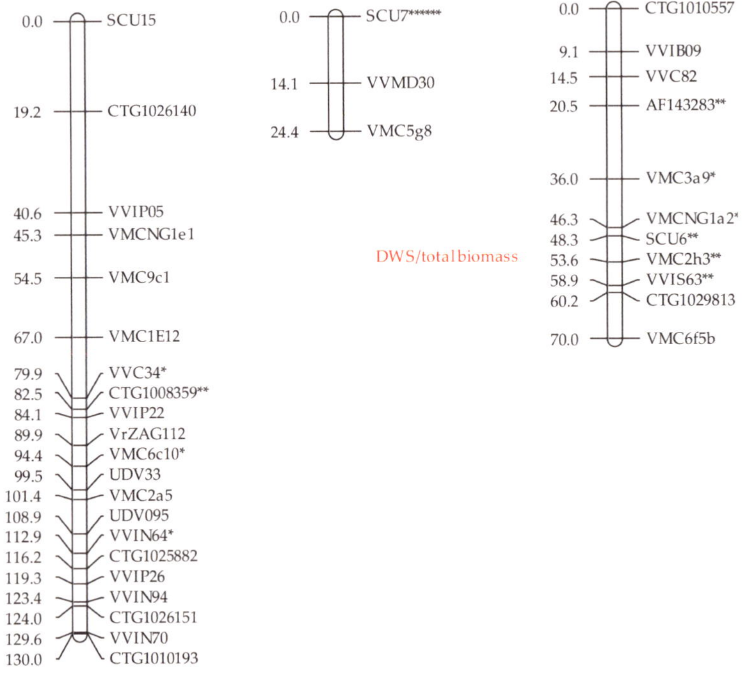

Figure 8.
Consensus linkage map from Ramsey and Riparia Gloire de Montpellier. Chromosomes 14, 15, and 17. In green, QTLs mapped in 2014. In red, QTLs mapped in 2015.

in chromosomes 3, 10, and 11 for canopy biomass (what we consider vigor), LA, and biomass partitioning (canopy/DWR).

Negative interaction was also found in chromosome 13 of Ramsey. LA/total biomass, LA/DWR, SLA, and DWS/total biomass were mapped in the parental map but were not found in the consensus map.

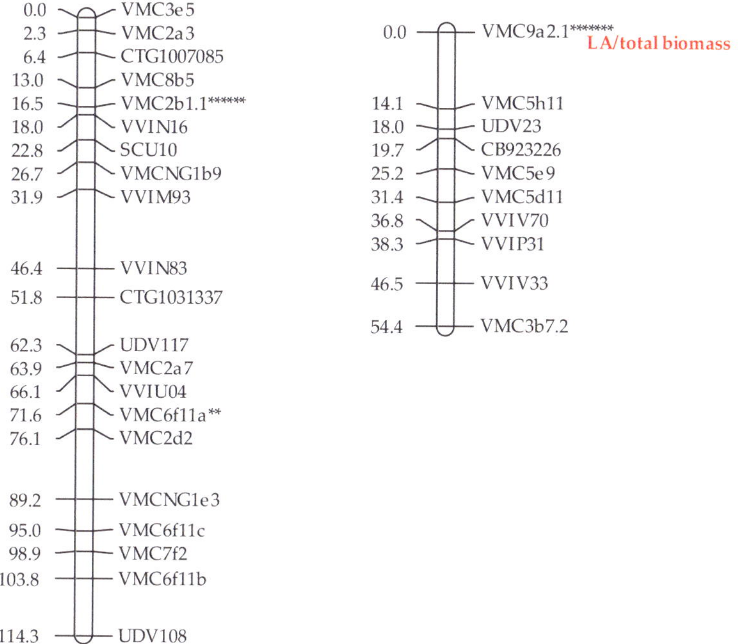

Figure 9.
Consensus linkage map from Ramsey and Riparia Gloire de Montpellier. Chromosomes 18 and 19. In red, in chromosome 19, the QTLs mapped in 2015.

With regard to the consensus map of 2015 (**Table 6**), many QTLs that were not mapped in 2014 were mapped this time. Six QTLs were found to be significant at the chromosome level, while only one was significant genome wide. In chromosome 19, one QTL for LA/total biomass, also found in Ramsey, explained 15% of total variance.

As observed in 2014, negative interaction was also found in 2015. This time, DWS, canopy, leaf number, growth rate, total biomass, canopy/DWR, DWR/DWS, SLA, DWS/DWL, and DWS/DWL were mapped in the parental map of Ramsey, but were not found in consensus map. The same happened for SLA and growth rate in reference to the *V. riparia* GM parental map that showed QTLs for these traits, but were not found in consensus.

Figures 4–9 show the linkage map of Ramsey and *V. riparia* GM [24], the 19 chromosomes and the approximate localization of the QTLs mapped in consensus maps. In green, QTLs were found in the first year, 2014. In red, QTLs were found in the second mapping, from 2015. QTL mapping was carried out with JoinMap/MapQTL 6 2003–2018, Kyazma B.V.

4. Identifying other quantitative traits in grapevine: QTL maps and underlying phenotypes

One major purpose in grapevine genetics is to identify quantitative loci, and underlying genes, that explain the natural genetic variation of specific traits. The frequent quantitative nature of genetic variation in grapevine requires the use of QTL mapping to understand the genetic architecture of traits. Several maps have been created and studied in grapevine with these purposes. Crosses between contrasting varieties have given birth to several progenies that constitute the basis for QTL/genetic mapping. Agronomic interesting traits like resistances to powdery and downy mildew, Phylloxera, Pierce's disease, and Xiphinema were studied in *V. vinifera* complex hybrids, *V. cinerea*, *V. rupestris*, and *V. arizonica* [30–37]. QTLs related to growth and development were found in progenies like Picovine × Ugni blanc [38], Riesling × Gewurztraminer [39], and Syrah and Grenache [40]. Also, in *V. vinifera* complex hybrids and *V. cinerea*, *V. rupestris*, and *V. arizonica*, traits related to plant physiology were studied: flowering and ripening dates, flower sex, and mineral deficiencies [21, 30–32, 41, 42]. Additionally, in Syrah × Pinot Noir, Grzeskowiak et al. [43] detected QTLs related to budburst, flowering beginning, the onset of ripening (*véraison*), and total fertility, while Bayo Canha [44] studied Monastrell × Syrah in search for QTLs related to phenology, enology-related traits, and productive and morphological traits.

Breeding purposes include a wide spectrum of objectives. Classic breeding programs have searched for biotic and abiotic resistances, as well as production, quality, growth, and developmental characteristics. Genomic studies and genetic mapping can significantly speed up the selection of seedlings with desired traits. Early identification of individuals carrying the desired allele combinations results in decreased maintenance and evaluation costs. The identification of genes and molecular markers underlying specific traits will help accelerate the breeding process, generating new prospects for crop improvement [44].

5. Conclusions

Vigor, a quantitative character, is particularly difficult to address. A large number of variables need to be studied in order to achieve a fine comprehension of the phenomena involved. In our study, we analyzed vigor from a wide physiological view and a genetic mapping approach. The mathematical function that represents growth, called sigmoid, starts with an initial plateau where small effects occur. Later, as these small effects accumulate, and cause successive effects, the function turns exponential. For quantitative characters, where positive feedbacks (typically exponential) can cause large effects, low but statistically significant explanatory levels, like the QTLs found, as well as the physiologic results, may have impressive effects.

It turns interesting to observe that many variables that physiologically showed to be significant in vigor explanation could be mapped and significant QTLs were found for them. The most important ones, SLA, LA, and LA/total biomass, showed to be significant in the PCA analysis as well as for the QTL mapping.

Previous studies bring support to our findings. When mapping the population of Picovine × Ugni blanc, Houel et al. [38] also found a QTL for LA in chromosome 4 of the parental map of ugni blanc and one QTL for LA in chromosome 9 of Picovine. In addition, QTLs related to budbreak explaining 11 and 12% of variation were mapped in chromosomes 4 and 19 in the Riesling × Gewurztraminer population [39], and five QTLs for growth rate were found in linkage groups 4, 10, 15, 17, and 18, in the Syrah and grenache population, altogether accounting for up to 30% of total variance [40]. Moreover, Díaz-Riquelme et al. [45] found that five MIKC genes (that encode for transcription factors with growth and developmental functions in plants) of grapevine were localized in chromosome 1. In our mapping, the major number of QTLs was found in chromosomes 1, 3, 5, 13, and 19, coincident with other studies.

After the QTL mapping, the next step would be to manage the search of candidate genes by saturating the portion of the chromosome that includes the interesting QTL and narrowing the piece of DNA that includes the candidate genes. As an example, by saturating chromosome 19, we could try to find candidate genes for the expression of the relation among LA and biomass production. This would finally support a breeding strategy, where to have a more efficient growing plant could turn to be important.

Vigor in grapevine, as many quantitative traits, appears to have a complex genetic background. This character, beside its biological significance, has a wide agronomical impact, not only related to the plant behavior but also linked to the amount and the quality of the harvest. In this paper, the analysis over a segregating progeny of Ramsey × *V. riparia* GM was able to identify several vigor-linked traits with good statistical support. Whereas the effect expected to be explained for each individual trait appears to be small, it will shed light to this complex character.

The phenotyping of segregating progenies constitutes a valuable tool for clarifying the genetic basis of traits of complex nature. An accurate choice of the parameters to be studied is crucial in order to optimize the experimental procedure and data analysis. In consequence, a previous understanding of the physiological basis of a trait of interest, or at least a very well-supported hypothesis, should lead a population genetics study. When these issues are considered, the obtained results would be able to achieve the expected goal.

Acknowledgements

Results shown in this Chapter were supported by INTA EEA Mendoza, Argentina and Viticulture and Enology, UC Davis, CA, USA.

We especially thank Nina Romero, Joaquín Fraga, Andy Viet Nguyen, Cassie Bent, Becky Wheeler, Karla Huerta, Jake Uretsky and Ashley Eustis for their valuable help in assessing and measuring experiments.

Author details

Inés Pilar Hugalde[1,2]*, Summaira Riaz[2], Cecilia B. Agüero[2], Hernán Vila[1], Sebastián Gomez Talquenca[1] and M. Andrew Walker[2]

1 Estación Experimental Agropecuaria Mendoza, INTA, Mendoza, Argentina

2 Department of Viticulture and Enology, UC Davis, Davis, CA, USA

*Address all correspondence to: hugalde.ines@inta.gob.ar

References

[1] Sax K. The association of size differences with seed-coat pattern and pigmentation in *Phaseolus vulgaris*. Genetics. 1923;**8**(6):552

[2] Thoday JM. Location of polygenes. Nature. 1960;**191**:368-370

[3] Torres AM et al. QTL detection and application to plant breeding. In: La genetica de los caracteres cuantitativos en al mejora vegetal del siglo XXI. España: Sociedad Espanola de Genetica; Sociedad Espanola de Ciencias Horticolas; 2012

[4] Donoso Contreras JM. Genética de la introgresión de genes del almendro (*Prunus dulcis* Mill.) en el melocotonero [*P. persica* (L.) Batsch]: desarrollo de una estrategia de selección de líneas casi isogénicas (Nils) con marcadores moleculares; 2014

[5] Falconer DS, Mackay TF, Frankham R. Introduction to quantitative genetics (4th ed). Trends in Genetics. 1996;**12**(7):280

[6] Lynch M, Walsh B. Genetics and Analysis of Quantitative Traits. Vol. 1. Massachusetts, USA: Sinauer Sunderland; 1998

[7] Lander ES, Botstein D. Mapping mendelian factors underlying quantitative traits using RFLP linkage maps. Genetics. 1989;**121**(1):185-199

[8] Jansen RC, Stam P. High resolution of quantitative traits into multiple loci via interval mapping. Genetics. 1994;**136**(4):1447-1455

[9] Boopathi NM. Marker-assisted selection. In: Genetic Mapping and Marker Assisted Selection. Springer; 2013. pp. 173-186

[10] Churchill GA, Doerge RW. Empirical threshold values for quantitative trait mapping. Genetics. 1994;**138**(3):963-971

[11] Ollat N et al. Vigour conferred by rootstock: Hypotheses and direction for research. Bulletin de l'OIV. 2003;**76**(869/870):581-595

[12] Rebolledo M et al. Phenotypic and genetic dissection of component traits for early vigour in rice using plant growth modelling, sugar content analyses and association mapping. Journal of Experimental Botany. 2015;**66**(18):5555-5566

[13] Wong SC, Cowan IR, Farquhar GD. Stomatal conductance correlates with photosynthetic capacity. Nature. 1979;**282**(5737):424

[14] Rogiers SY et al. Stomatal response of an anisohydric grapevine cultivar to evaporative demand, available soil moisture and abscisic acid. Tree Physiology. 2012;**32**(3):249-261

[15] Polymenis M, Schmidt EV. Coupling of cell division to cell growth by translational control of the G1 cyclin CLN3 in yeast. Genes & Development. 1997;**11**(19):2522-2531

[16] Cosgrove DJ. Growth of the plant cell wall. Nature Reviews Molecular Cell Biology. 2005;**6**(11):850-861

[17] De Herralde F et al. Effects of rootstock and irrigation regime on hydraulic architecture of *Vitis vinifera* L. cv. tempranillo. Journal International des Sciences de la Vigne et du Vin. 2006;**40**(3):133-139

[18] Lovisolo C et al. An abscisic acid-related reduced transpiration promotes gradual embolism repair when grapevines are rehydrated after drought. New Phytologist. 2008;**180**(3):642-651

[19] Di Filippo M, Vila H. Influence of different rootstocks on the vegetative and reproductive performance of *Vitis vinifera* L. malbec under irrigated conditions. Journal International des Sciences de la Vigne et du Vin. 2011;**45**(2):75-84

[20] Keller M. The Science of Grapevines: Anatomy and Physiology. Prosser, WA, USA: Academic Press; 2015

[21] Marguerit E et al. Rootstock control of scion transpiration and its acclimation to water deficit are controlled by different genes. New Phytologist. 2012;**194**(2):416-429

[22] Adam-Blondon A-F et al. Mapping 245 SSR markers on the *Vitis vinifera* genome: A tool for grape genetics. Theoretical and Applied Genetics. 2004;**109**(5):1017-1027

[23] Riaz S et al. A microsatellite marker based framework linkage map of *Vitis vinifera* L. Theoretical and Applied Genetics. 2004;**108**(5):864-872

[24] Lowe K, Walker M. Genetic linkage map of the interspecific grape rootstock cross Ramsey (*Vitis champinii*) × Riparia Gloire (*Vitis riparia*). Theoretical and Applied Genetics. 2006;**112**(8):1582-1592

[25] Hugalde I et al. Physiological and Genetic Control of Vigour in A 'Ramsey' × 'Riparia Gloire de Montpellier' Population. Leuven, Belgium: International Society for Horticultural Science (ISHS); 2017

[26] Lovisolo C et al. Expression of PIP1 and PIP2 aquaporins is enhanced in olive dwarf genotypes and is related to root and leaf hydraulic conductance. Physiologia Plantarum. 2007;**130**(4):543-551

[27] Kaldenhoff R et al. Significance of plasmalemma aquaporins for water-transport in Arabidopsis thaliana. The Plant Journal. 1998;**14**(1):121-128

[28] Clearwater M, Lowe R, Hofstee B, Barclay C, Mandemaker A, Blattmann P. Hydraulic conductance and rootstock effects in grafted vines of kiwifruit. Journal of experimental botany. 2004;55:1371-1382

[29] Sivasakthi K et al. Chickpea genotypes contrasting for vigor and canopy conductance also differ in their dependence on different water transport pathways. Frontiers in Plant Science. 2017;**8**:1663

[30] Dalbó M et al. Marker-assisted selection for powdery mildew resistance in grapes. Journal of the American Society for Horticultural Science. 2001;**126**(1):83-89

[31] Fischer BM et al. Quantitative trait locus analysis of fungal disease resistance factors on a molecular map of grapevine. Theoretical and Applied Genetics. 2004;**108**(3):501-515

[32] Welter LJ et al. Genetic mapping and localization of quantitative trait loci affecting fungal disease resistance and leaf morphology in grapevine (*Vitis vinifera* L.). Molecular Breeding. 2007;**20**(4):359-374

[33] Krivanek A, Riaz S, Walker M. Identification and molecular mapping of PdR1, a primary resistance gene to Pierce's disease in *Vitis*. Theoretical and Applied Genetics. 2006;**112**(6):1125-1131

[34] Riaz S et al. Fine-scale genetic mapping of two Pierce's disease resistance loci and a major segregation distortion region on chromosome 14 of grape. Theoretical and Applied Genetics. 2008;**117**(5):671

[35] Riaz S et al. Refined mapping of the Pierce's disease resistance locus, PdR1, and sex on an extended genetic map of *Vitis rupestris* × *V. arizonica*. Theoretical and Applied Genetics. 2006;**113**(7):1317

[36] Roush TL, Granett J, Walker MA. Inheritance of gall formation relative to phylloxera resistance levels in hybrid grapevines. American Journal of Enology and Viticulture. 2007;**58**(2):234-241

[37] Xu K et al. Genetic and QTL analysis of resistance to *Xiphinema index* in a grapevine cross. Theoretical and Applied Genetics. 2008;**116**(2):305-311

[38] Houel C et al. Identification of stable QTLs for vegetative and reproductive traits in the microvine (*Vitis vinifera* L.) using the 18 K Infinium chip. BMC Plant Biology. 2015;**15**(1):1

[39] Duchêne E et al. Towards the adaptation of grapevine varieties to climate change: QTLs and candidate genes for developmental stages. Theoretical and Applied Genetics. 2012;**124**(4):623-635

[40] Coupel-Ledru A et al. Reduced nighttime transpiration is a relevant breeding target for high water-use efficiency in grapevine. Proceedings of the National Academy of Sciences. 2016;**113**(32):8963-8968

[41] Mandl K et al. A genetic map of Welschriesling × Sirius for the identification of magnesium-deficiency by QTL analysis. Euphytica. 2006;**149**(1-2):133-144

[42] Costantini L et al. Berry and phenology-related traits in grapevine (*Vitis vinifera* L.): From quantitative trait loci to underlying genes. BMC Plant Biology. 2008;**8**(1):38

[43] Grzeskowiak L et al. Candidate loci for phenology and fruitfulness contributing to the phenotypic variability observed in grapevine. Theoretical and Applied Genetics. 2013;**126**(11):2763-2776

[44] Bayo Canha A. Genetic Analysis of Traits of Interest in *Vitis vinifera* Using a Progeny of Wine Grapes. PhD thesis. Universidad Politécnica de Cartagena. Colombia: Monastrell x Syrah; 2015

[45] Díaz-Riquelme J et al. Genome-wide analysis of MIKCC-type MADS box genes in grapevine. Plant Physiology. 2009;**149**(1):354-369

Section 3

Genetic Diversity in Crop Management

Chapter 3

Weedy Rice: Competitive Ability, Evolution, and Diversity

Swati Shrestha, Shandrea Stallworth and Te-Ming Tseng

Abstract

Weedy rice is conspecific, the most troublesome weed of cultivated rice identified as a threat to global rice production. The weed has inherited high reproductive ability and high dormancy by outcrossing with modern rice cultivars and wild cultivars, respectively. Traits such as rapid growth, high tillering, enhanced ability to uptake fertilizers, asynchronous maturation, seed shattering, and long dormancy periods make weedy rice more competitive than cultivated rice. Weedy rice infesting rice fields are morphologically diverse with different hull color, awn length, plant height, and variable tiller number. Morphological diversity in weedy rice can be attributed to its high genetic diversity. Introgression of alleles from cultivated rice into weedy has resulted in high genetic and morphological diversity in weedy rice. Although variations among weedy rice populations make them difficult to control, on the brighter side, competitive nature of weedy rice could be considered as raw genetic materials for rice breeding program to develop vigorous rice plants able to tolerate high biotic and abiotic stresses.

Keywords: genetic diversity, phenotypic diversity, rice breeding, red rice, abiotic stress tolerance, biotic stress tolerance

1. Introduction

Weedy rice, also called as red rice because of its red pericarp, belongs to same genus and species as the cultivated rice, *Oryza sativa* L. It is one of the major weeds in rice field worldwide [1] and adulterates cultivated rice decreasing its productivity in the field and reducing crop quality due to seed contamination. Rice monocropping and direct-seeded rice system promote infestation of weedy rice, and severe infestation of weedy rice can cause up to 100% yield reduction in direct-seeded rice system [2]. Numerous weed control strategies are adopted by the farmers to control weedy rice in rice fields. Development of herbicide-tolerant rice was thought to solve the problem of weedy rice, but with the development of herbicide-resistant weeds, the value of this technology has become questionable. Management of weedy rice in rice fields is possible only through adoption of integrated weed management practice such as winter flooding, fallow tillage, and crop rotation [3].

The genus *Oryza* has 21 wild and two cultivated species. Two cultivated species include *O. sativa* the Asian rice and *O. glaberrima* the African rice, both with diploid AA genome. *O. sativa* has three major subspecies: *indica*, *japonica*, and *javanica*. Among the wild rice, nine are tetraploid (BBCC) (CCDD) and 12 are diploid [4]. Wild rice found in nature are those derived from *O. sativa*

(AA complex) and *O. Officinalis* complex (BB, CC, CCDD) [5]. *Oryza sativa* complex includes *O. rufipogon*, *O. barthii*, and *O. longistaminata*, while *O. officinalis* complex includes *O. punctata*, *O. latifolia*, and *O. officinalis.* However, weedy rice is distinct from wild rice and is believed to have been evolved through (i) hybridization among and within cultivated and wild rice, (ii) de-domestication of cultivated rice, and (iii) direct colonization of wild rice in agricultural rice fields [6].

The genus *Oryza* consists of numerous species, and studying the genetic structure of cultivated, wild, and weedy rice species is crucial for understanding the morphological and physiological characters of rice cultivars and the genes governing these characters. Proper understanding of numerous genes governing quantitative and qualitative traits in rice is essential for successful molecular breeding programs. Genetic diversity of *Oryza* can be utilized for crop improvement program by plant breeders in order to produce rice cultivars with higher yield that could meet the growing food demand.

2. Weedy rice: a troublesome weed

Weedy rice (*Oryza sativa spp.) is* currently distributed worldwide, and it is known to infest the areas in and around rice fields [7]. These weedy rice tend to have many undesirable traits when compared to cultivated rice such as the ability to germinate faster, reduce yields by 90%, and persist within the soil bed for up to 10 years [8]. Conventionally, in most of the developing countries, rice is transplanted into standing water, thus providing competitive advantage to the crop and enhancing crop productivity by suppressing weeds [9]. However, with the scarcity of labor and water, there has been a significant shift from puddled transplanting (PTR) to direct-seeded rice (DSR) system in Asian countries in the past two decades [2]. In the USA, all rice fields are cultivated through highly mechanized DSR system [10]. DSR involves rice stand establishment directly by sowing seeds in the fields and uses less water and labor and emits less methane than the PTR system [11]. Although DSR has numerous advantages over the PTR, sustainability of DSR with reference to control of weedy rice is becoming questionable. Currently, weedy rice has been reported in most of the rice-growing countries like China, India, the USA, Bangladesh, Bhutan, Brazil, Nepal, Thailand, Japan, the Philippines, Korea, Thailand, Sri Lanka, Vietnam, and Malaysia (**Figure 1**) [15]. Incidence of weedy rice has increased tremendously in Malaysia following the adoption of DSR in the 1980s [12]. In Vietnam, yield loss due to weedy rice has been reported from 15 to 70% [13]. Due to its ability to behave similarly to rice, management of these weedy species without causing damage to the crop itself has proven to be an issue [14].

According to Allston, the first weedy red rice was reported in the USA as early as 1800 as seed contaminants from Asia and since then has been affecting rice crop by limiting its yield [16]. Weedy rice share common gene pool with cultivated rice making them morphologically similar to cultivated rice but have high seed shattering and differential dormancy, making them difficult to control weeds in the rice fields. Some of the unfavorable traits possessed by weedy rice are long culm lengths, high tillering capacity, light leaf color, weak culms, red pericarp, highly shattering seeds, and high degree of seed dormancy [2, 17, 18]. It is difficult to control weedy rice because they mimic cultivated rice morphologically, biochemically, and physiologically. Physical weed management is difficult as weedy rice is morphologically similar to cultivated rice in early stages, and chemical weed management is limited as herbicides controlling weedy rice also kill rice plant [2]. In many places, farmers have altered their cropping pattern to non-rice system to manage this noxious weed [14]. Depending on the amount of infestation, weedy rice can cause yield losses

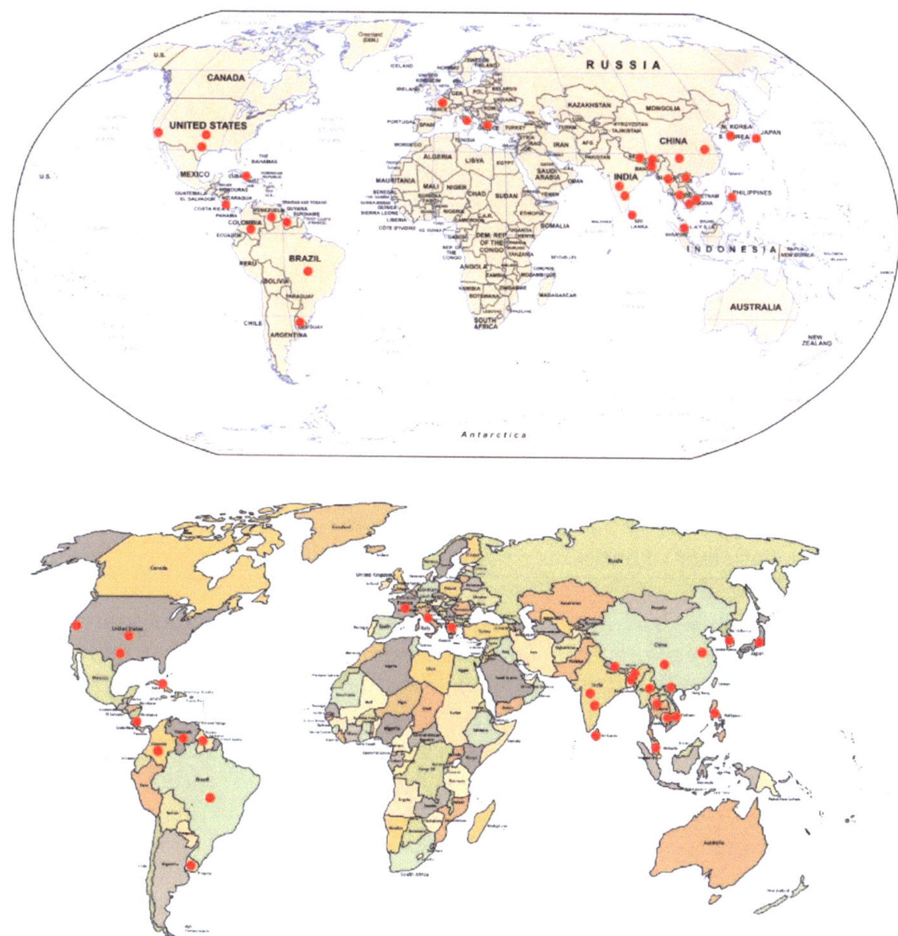

Figure 1.
Weedy rice distribution worldwide. Red dots represent regions where weedy rice infestation has been reported [15].

varying from 50 to 60% under moderate infestation to 70–80% under heavy infestation. In Arkansas, the highest rice-producing state in the USA, economic loss due to weedy rice has been estimated to be $274/hectare [19]. The threshold for weedy rice infestation is one to three plants/m^2 in the USA; plant density higher than this can cause significant yield loss [20].

3. Competitive nature of weedy rice

Competition for limited resource is the drawing force for natural selection and shaping plant communities [21]. Weeds compete with crop for nutrients, space, and light, thus decreasing yield potential of crop. Traits of weedy rice such as taller growth habit, higher tillering, and higher nutrient use efficiency make it dominant and more competitive than the crop [22]. The success of weedy rice as weeds can be attributed to its high dormancy as they can remain viable in soil for a long period of time and emerge when conditions are favorable [23]. Noldin et al., in 2006, conducted an experiment to evaluate the dormancy and longevity of various weedy rice biotypes from four states in the USA [24]. The study found the differential level of dormancy among weedy rice ecotypes buried under the soil at different depths, and all of them were more viable than commercial rice cultivar. Five weedy ecotypes had viable seeds even after 36 months of burial in the soil. The commercial rice seeds were nonviable after 5 months of burial in the soil. Weedy rice therefore has greater viability than cultivated rice under certain environmental conditions and can emerge from deeper soil surface, thus developing a robust soil seedbank [24].

Seed shattering, which distinguishes cultivated rice from its wild forms, is variable in weedy rice [25]. In weedy rice, the abscission layer degrades earlier as compared to cultivated rice, leading to earlier shattering and increasing its fitness for survival in the environment [26]. Shattering in weedy rice is controlled by unidentified regulatory genes distinct from wild rice, thus suggesting parallel evolution between weedy rice and wild rice [26]. Weedy rice is also generally taller than cultivated rice making them more efficient for light and space [27]. Weedy rice has higher nitrogen use efficiency causing greater yield loss in rice fields [28]. Thus, in fields infested with weedy rice, the application of nitrogen fertilizers may not lead to an eventual increase in rice yields; instead, the weedy rice plants grow bigger and compete more aggressively with rice resulting in rice plants with lower yield [28]. Nitrogen accumulation is higher in weedy rice than in cultivated rice in "nutrient-deficient" conditions, suggesting a more efficient nutrient uptake mechanism in weedy rice than cultivated rice [29]. In addition to higher nutrient response, weedy rice also has higher stress tolerance [30, 31]. Unlike commercial rice varieties, weedy rice can perform better in unfavorable environmental conditions such as higher carbon dioxide, lower nutrient supply, and high/low temperature, indicating that they have higher capability of enduring stress than cultivated rice and, therefore, thrive better in stressful environment. Weedy rice ecotypes have higher leaf area and root weight when grown at carbon dioxide level of 500 μmol mol^{-1} which is the projected CO_2 concentration in the middle and end of the twentieth century [30]. In saline conditions, growth and germination of most plant species are reduced; however, weedy rice accessions have higher germination index and seedling vigor than commercial rice at 16 dSm^{-1} (NaCl) salinity level [32]. A weed-crop competition modeled by Pantone and Baker showed that weedy rice is more dominant than cultivated rice and competitive ability of one weedy rice plant is equivalent to three plants of an old commercial rice variety "Mars" [33]. Ottis et al. studied the interference potential of weedy rice on five rice cultivars (CL161, Cocodrie, LaGrue, Lemont, and XL8) and demonstrated that yield reduction of rice cultivars ranged from 100 to 755 kg/ha for every weedy rice plant/m^2 [34].

4. Evolution of weedy rice

There is immense diversity both among and within weedy rice populations and between weedy and cultivated rice [35–38]. Studying the differences in weedy rice populations in relation to phenological and morphological traits will help us better understand the evolution of weedy traits. There are a number of hypotheses that speak to the origination of weedy rice. These hypotheses include the following: weedy rice is a crop mimic of rice similar to a wild relative, it is a hybrid of natural crosses between wild and cultivated rice, and it is merely an evolved taxon from cultivated rice [39]. In areas inhabited by wild rice, De-Wet and Harlan believed that weedy rice arose from the selection of wild rice to agricultural habits for consumption [40]. While this may be true for areas with a prominent wild rice population, it does not address the prevalence of this weedy species in areas uninhabited by wild rice. Recent genetic studies point to specific examples of the evolutionary pathways of weedy rice.

Over the last 20 years, studies conducted on weedy rice have increased due to the increased infestation in rice fields. In 2006, Cao et al. noticed the resurgence of weedy rice and set out to conduct a molecular study utilizing 20 simple sequence repeat (SSR) markers and 30 different populations of weedy rice to identify the evolution of weeds in China's Liaoning province [41]. The weedy rice populations were compared to a wild rice relative, *O. rufipogon*, as well as cultivars to represent both indica and japonica biotypes. Cao et al. discovered, through genetic data, that the Liaoning cultivar, a japonica biotype, was very similar to that of weedy rice and clustered together to demonstrate this, while another Chinese japonica biotype did not follow the same clustering style. Through AMOVA analysis, the study found approximately 35% of the total genetic variation among regions, 18% within regions, and 46% within the populations. When the wild relative, *O. rufipogon*, and indica biotypes were compared to the weeds, they were further clustered from the weedy rice and Liaoning cultivar. Based on this data and the clusters presented, the authors concluded that weedy rice in the Liaoning province of China arose from the mutation and hybridization of Liaoning rice varieties [41]. This conclusion was challenged in 2010 by a paper from Ellstrand et al. stating "...if hybridization had occurred, it is likely that some *O. rufipogon* alleles would have been retained in the weedy lineages in the short time that they have been problematic" [38]. This could be true as Cao et al. found that there was a lack of heterozygosity within the weedy rice populations.

Weedy rice can also be referred to as red rice due to the presence of a red pericarp not often witnessed within the cultivated rice. To determine if the presence of a red pericarp was a characteristic of weedy rice or cultivated rice, Gealy et al. used SSR markers to differentiate between weedy rice present in the Southeastern USA, cultivated rice, and hybrids [42]. In this study, 31 SSR markers were used to analyze 180 kinds of rice from the genus *Oryza* and 80 weedy rice and rice cultivars from the USA. The 31 SSR markers selected represented low to high polymorphism information content values to screen the population for genetic variation. Using AMOVA, the genetic variation of the 80 weedy rice and rice cultivars was 56% within populations and 44% among populations. When the study compared only the 38 weedy rice populations that were separated into three different weedy rice populations, the genetic variation was 47% within populations and 53% among populations. A large amount of genetic variability was explained by the considerable genetic variation within blackhull, awned red rice (BA+), and *Oryza sativa* with white bran (OSW). Gealy et al. also found that when comparing hull types among the red rice population, red rice with straw or blackhulls and awns were not molecularly different from one another. Gealy et al. found that many of the SSR markers used were able to differentiate between the OSW and the weedy rice. There were 12 SSR markers that produced alleles that were present in the cultivated rice with white bran that was absent in the weedy rice populations [42]. Through the study, they found that BA+ weedy rice had a greater genetic distance and more diversity than its strawhull, awnless counterparts with both varying genetically from the historic OSW population. To understand these differences, Gealy et al. also used principal component analysis to look at the clustering of populations based on genetic distance [43]. Through the analysis, they were able to find that hybrids were more closely associated with the weedy rice parent. This data was closely related to earlier studies completed by Gealy et al. [43]. Using structure analysis, genetic structure groupings were used to visualize the genetic backgrounds of weedy rice present in the USA. Six different groups were identified using STRUCTURE software by Pritchard et al. [44]. When analyzing the weedy rice population, the hybrid weedy rice fell in between strawhull, awnless and blackhull, awned weedy rice. This outcome was expected given the data presented on genetic variation and principal component analysis. The same results were observed when all rice in the study were combined together suggesting that the selected SSR markers by Gealy et al. were able to capture enough genetic variability to differentiate the origination of sampled weedy rice present within the USA [42]. Gealy et al. went further and compared their findings to those of Cao et al. notating that US weedy rice was qualitatively different from those found in the Liaoning province of China. While US weedy rice was genetically different from historical rice grown in the USA, they were more closely related to *O. sativa*, *nivara*, or *rufipogon* species, but Liaoning weedy rice populations were related to rice grown in the area and *japonica* biotypes from other regions [42]. These findings could be related to the selection of SSR markers used in the study by Cao et al. lacking the ability to capture as much genetic variation present in their population [42]. While Gealy et al. used 31 SSR markers and Cao et al. used 20 SSR markers, the quality of markers may not have been to the same degree as Gealy et al.

5. Weedy rice diversity

5.1 Morphological diversity of weedy rice

Weedy rice exhibits high genetic and phenotypic diversity, and this diversity is dependent on the ecotype and habitat [45]. Weedy rice from different regions of Asia (Malaysia, the Philippines, Thailand, and Vietnam) varied in terms of grain characteristics and growth response under competition with cultivated rice [46]. The Philippines weedy rice produced the highest grain yield, while a higher growth potential was observed in weedy rice from Vietnam; weedy rice from Thailand was the shortest. Weedy rice from major rice-growing areas of Ampara District, Sri Lanka, were found to be morphologically diverse in terms of tiller number, plant height, and panicle number [47]. In Peninsular Malaysia, the weedy rice can be divided into four major clusters based on their morphological variation: (1) awned black and brownhull derived from wild *Oryza* population, (2) strawhull awnless weedy rice derived from rice cultivars with high shattering, (3) brownhull weedy rice, and (4) weedy rice of mixed weedy morphotype inferring multiple origin [48]. Similarly, weedy rice from major rice-cultivating areas of Italy can be awned, awnless, or mucronate. The highest variability was observed among awned weedy rice ecotypes than the awnless in terms of flag leaf length, 1000 seed weight, and germination rates [49]. In Arkansas, morphological characteristics varied among the two weedy rice ecotypes and within each ecotype (**Figure 2**) [45]. Blackhull weedy rice ecotype showed greater variation in traits than strawhull weedy rice. Plant height among blackhull accessions ranged from as short as 75 cm to as tall as 190 cm. The range of plant height in strawhull was greater (46–189 cm), but on an average, they were slightly shorter than blackhull weedy rice. Flag leaf lengths were longer in strawhull, 38 cm, than in blackhull weedy rice, 34 cm. Tillering capacity of blackhull weedy rice (mean = 105 tillers per plant) was higher than strawhull (mean = 95 tillers per plant). Also, weedy rice accessions from northeastern region of Arkansas flowered earlier than other regions in Arkansas. As the weedy rice is conspecific species of rice with AA genome, it has traits of both cultivated and wild rice. Weedy rice, being closely related to cultivated rice, has a tendency to pollinate with cultivated rice and produce progeny of different phenotypes [50]. Thus, weedy rice all over the world have

DOI: http://dx.doi.org/10.5772/intechopen.81838

variable phenotype as they can readily exchange genetic information with nearby cultivated rice plants.

5.2 Genetic diversity of weedy rice and its gene flow potential

Morphological diversity in weedy rice can be attributed to its high genetic diversity. The genetic diversity of rice has been estimated using various markers like random amplified polymorphic DNA (RAPD), restriction fragment length polymorphism (RFLP), amplified fragment length polymorphism (AFLP), and simple sequence repeats (SSR) [50–54]. Of these SSR markers are most commonly

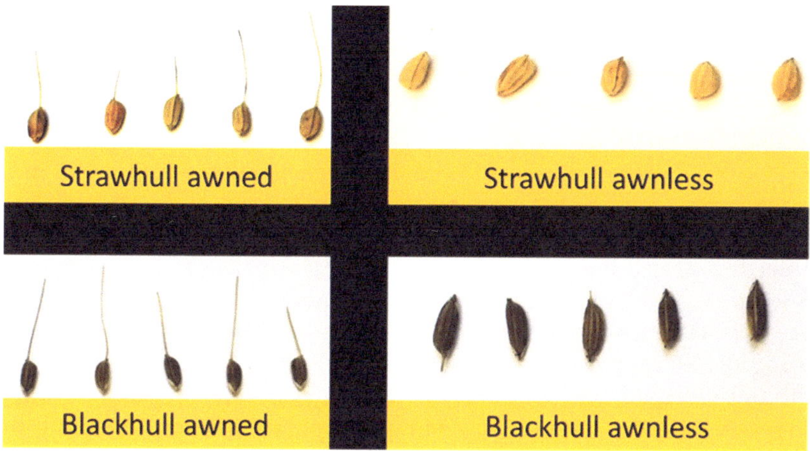

Figure 2.
Weedy rice of different hull color and awn length collected from various rice fields of Arkansas, USA, in 2008–2009.

Species	Geographical location	Marker used	Genetic diversity	Reference
Oryza sativa f. *spontanea*	Northeastern China	SSR	Heterozygosity (H_e) = 0.313 Shannon's diversity index (I) = 0.572	Cao et al. [41]
Oryza sativa L.	Northeast Asia	SSR	H_e = 0.748 I = 0.434	Mao-bai et al. [51]
Oryza sativa L.	Liaoning province, China	SSR	H_e = 0.053	Yu et al. [52]
Awnless red rice	Arkansas, USA	SSR	Average genetic distance = 0.2	Gealy et al. [59]
Awned red rice	Arkansas, USA	SSR	Average genetic distance = 0.33	Gealy et al. [59]
Oryza sativa	Arkansas, USA	SSR	Nei's genetic distance (GD) = 0.7	Shivrain et al. [54]
Oryza sativa L.	Italy	SSR	H_e = 0.295	Grimm et al. [56]
Red rice	Uruguay	AFLP	Average of 25.6 bands per primer pair	Federici et al. [57]

Table 1.
Genetic diversity of weedy rice (Oryza sativa) from different regions of the world as detected by molecular markers.

used as they are readily available, easy to use, highly polymorphic, and less expensive and give accurate results (**Table 1**). Genetic diversity of weedy rice populations from Liaoning province using SSR markers was found to be relatively high with H_e value of 0.313, and 35% of genetic variation was among regions [41]. Weedy rice from Northeast Asia are genetically diverse with high Shannon's information index of 0.748 and heterozygosity of 0.434 [51]. Among RAPD and SSR markers, SSR were superior to RAPD in detecting genetic diversity among weedy rice populations [52]. Weedy rice, weedy rice-cultivated rice hybrids, and rice cultivars can be distinguished using microsatellite SSR markers [53]. Molecular studies using SSR confirmed the differentiation of the two weedy rice ecotypes from Arkansas, USA [54]. Strawhull weedy rice were genetically distant compared to blackhull weedy rice. A higher genetic diversity within blackhull weedy rice (D = 0.76) was estimated compared to strawhull (D = 0.68). US weedy rice has high genetic diversity with nucleotide diversity (Pi) = 1.48 per Kb, thus indicating their higher potential to evolve [54]. Within weedy rice populations, the blackhull group showed higher nucleotide diversity (Pi = 0.66) than strawhull group (Pi = 0.56). Weedy rice was found to be closely related to *O. sativa* indica and *O. sativa* aus, instead of the commonly cultivated rice in the USA, *O. sativa* japonica [55]. Similar results were also observed by Londo and Schaal where most of the weedy rice clustered together with *O. sativa* aus. These results suggest that the US weedy rice evolved from *O. sativa* indica and aus rather than *O. sativa* japonica [38]. Genetic diversity of weedy rice from major rice-growing areas of Italy using 19 SSR markers was found to be relatively high with heterozygosity of 0.295 and average alleles of 3.368 [56]. Weedy rice from Uruguay is grouped into three distinct clusters based on their geographical location indicating similar characteristics of plants from similar location [57]. Great diversity in weedy rice accessions from different parts of the world supports the hypothesis that these are derived from natural hybridization among and within the cultivated and wild rice. It should be noted that not all blackhull, brownhull, and strawhull accessions are similar in terms of their genetic makeup or morphology. Their distinct characteristics can significantly affect management strategies that are adopted for controlling weedy rice making the control of weedy rice difficult.

Weedy rice and cultivated rice being closely related to each other have chances of exchanging genetic information. Gene flow from wild species to crop and vice versa has increasing practical implication with development of herbicide-resistant and genetically engineered crops. Transfer of genes conferring biotic and abiotic stress tolerance in crops to the wild species may pose great ecological threat. Thus, gene flow frequency between weedy rice and rice cultivars should be kept in mind while using weedy rice species for rice improvement programs. Studies have shown noticeable gene flow potential between weedy rice, wild rice, and cultivated rice. Gene flow frequency between weedy rice and cultivated rice ranged from 0.011 to 0.046% and between wild rice and cultivated rice ranged from 1.21 to 2.19% approximately [50]. Gene flow frequency from cultivated rice to wild rice (*O. rufipogon*) can be as high as 2.94% [58]. However, most of the gene flow studies have revealed outcrossing rate of up to 1% in *Oryza* species [59]. The variation in gene flow frequency in different studies reveals that the rate of gene flow between cultivated rice and their wild relatives depends upon various factors like weather conditions, density of infestation, and flowering synchrony. Studies have shown a possibility of crop-to-wild gene flow between *Oryza* species. As the infestation of weedy rice is increasing with change in rice production systems and climate change, the problem can become more severe in the future. Thus, steps should be taken to control weedy rice in the rice field, or it might have negative impacts on crop yield as well as the ecology of the area.

6. Conclusions

The research discussed above shows that weedy rice is one of the most successful weeds in rice due to key weedy traits including high seed dormancy and longevity, high seed shattering, high nutrient uptake and nitrogen use efficiency, more tillers, high panicle number and biomass, and tolerance to stresses including herbicides. For successful implementation of management strategies for weedy rice, the physiological and genetic basis of these competitive traits needs to be understood. Further, understanding the mechanism and genetic basis of these competitive traits may provide unique information for rice improvement owing to its close relationship with cultivated rice. However, numerous pros and cons associated with the use of the wild relatives for crop improvement program should be considered before using weedy rice as raw genetic material for developing robust rice cultivars.

Acknowledgements

This work is supported by the National Institute of Food and Agriculture, US Department of Agriculture, and Hatch Projects under accession number 230060 and is a contribution of the Mississippi Agricultural and Forestry Experiment Station.

Conflict of interest

The authors declare that this work was presented in the absence of any commercial or financial relationships that could be construed as a potential conflict of interest.

Author details

Swati Shrestha, Shandrea Stallworth and Te-Ming Tseng*
Mississippi State University, Mississippi State, Mississippi, USA

*Address all correspondence to: t.tseng@msstate.edu

References

[1] Norsworthy JK, Bond J, Scott RC. Weed management practices and needs in Arkansas and Mississippi rice. Weed Technology. 2013;**27**:623-630. DOI: 10.1614/WT-D-12-00172.1

[2] Ziska LH, Gealy DR, Burgos N, Caicedo AL, Gressel J, Lawton-Rauh AL, et al. Weedy (red) rice: An emerging constraint to global rice production. Advances in Agronomy. 2015;**129**:181-228. DOI: 10.1016/bs.agron.2014.09.003

[3] Burgos NR, Shivrain VK, Scott RC, Mauromoustakos A, Kuk YI, Sales MA, et al. Differential tolerance of weedy red rice (*Oryza sativa* L.) from Arkansas, USA to glyphosate. Crop Protection. 2011;**30**:986-994. DOI: 10.1016/j.cropro.2011.03.024

[4] Khush GS. Origin, dispersal, cultivation and variation of rice. Plant Molecular Biology. 2002;**35**:25-34. DOI: 10.1023/A:1005810616885

[5] Singh K, Kumar V, Saharawat YS, Gathala M, Ladha JK, Chauhan BS. Weedy rice: An emerging threat for direct-seeded rice production systems in India. Rice Research. 2013;**1**(1):1000106. DOI: 10.4172/jrr.1000106

[6] Kanapeckas KL, Vigueira CC, Ortiz A, Gettler KA, Burgos NR, Fischer AJ, et al. Escape to ferality: The endoferal origin of weedy rice from crop rice through de-domestication. PLoS One. 2016;**11**(9):e0162676. DOI: 10.1371/journal.pone.0162676

[7] Nadir S, Xiong H-B, Zhu Q, Zhang X-L, Xu H-Y, Li J, et al. Weedy rice in sustainable rice production. A review. Agronomy for Sustainable Development. 2017;**37**:1-14. DOI: 10.1007/s13593-017-0456-4

[8] Ferrero A. Weedy Rice, Biological Features and Control. FAO Plant Production and Protection Paper (FAO); 2003

[9] Muthayya S, Sugimoto JD, Montgomery S, Maberly GF. An overview of global rice production, supply, trade, and consumption. Annals of the New York Academy of Sciences. 2014;**1324**:7-14. DOI: 10.1111/nyas.12540

[10] Akita S. Direct rice-seeding culture in the United States. Farming Japan. 1991;**26**:20-26

[11] Liu H, Hussain S, Zheng M, Peng S, Huang J, Cui K, et al. Dry direct-seeded rice as an alternative to transplanted-flooded rice in Central China. Agronomy for Sustainable Development. 2015;**35**:285-294. DOI: 10.1007/s13593-014-0239-0

[12] Vaughan DA, Sanchez PL, Ushiki J, Kaga A, Tomooka N. Asian rice and weedy rice–evolutionary perspectives. In: Crop Ferality and Volunteerism. Boca Raton, USA: CRC Press; 2005. pp. 257-277

[13] Chin DV. Weedy rice situation in Vietnam. In: FAO Report. Global Workshop on Red Rice Control. Varadero, Cuba: Food and Agricultural Organization; 1999. pp. 67-74

[14] Chauhan BS. Strategies to manage weedy rice in Asia. Crop Protection. 2013;**48**:51-56. DOI: 10.1016/j.cropro.2013.02.015

[15] Chen LJ, Suh HS. Weedy rice—Origin and Dissemination. China: Yunnan Science and Technology Press; 2015. p. 234

[16] Allston RF. The rice plant. University of Michigan Humanities Text Initiative. 1846;**1**:320-256

[17] Tseng TM, Burgos NR, Alcober EAL, Shivrain VK. Inter- and intrapopulation variation in dormancy of *Oryza sativa* L. (weedy red rice) and

allelic variation of dormancy-linked loci. Weed Research. 2013;**53**:440-451. DOI: 10.1111/wre.12044

[18] Tseng TM, Shivrain VK, Lawton-Rauh A, Burgos NR. Dormancy-linked population structure of weedy rice (*Oryza sativa*). Weed Science. 2017;**66**:331-339. DOI: 10.1017/wsc.2017.86

[19] Burgos NR, Norsworthy JK, Scott RC, Smith KL. Red rice (*Oryza sativa*) status after 5 years of imidazolinone-resistant rice technology in Arkansas. Weed Technology. 2008;**22**:200-208. DOI: 10.1614/WT-07-075.1

[20] Smith RJ Jr. Weed thresholds in southern US rice, *Oryza sativa*. Weed Technology. 1988;**2**:232-241. DOI: 10.1017/S0890037X00030505

[21] Whittaker RH. Dominance and diversity in land plant communities: Numerical relations of species express the importance of competition in community function and evolution. Science. 1965;**147**:250-260. DOI: 10.1126/science.147.3655.250

[22] Estorninos LE Jr, Gealy DR, Talbert RE. Growth response of Rice (*Oryza sativa*) and red Rice (*O. sativa*) in a replacement series study. Weed Technology. 2002;**16**:401-406. DOI: 10.1614/0890-037X(2002)016[0401:GROROS]2.0.CO;2

[23] Goss WL, Brown E. Buried red rice seed. Journal of the American Society of Agronomy. 1939;**31**:633-637. ISSN: 0095-965

[24] Noldin JA, Chandler JM, McCauley GN. Seed longevity of red rice ecotypes buried in soil. Planta Daninha. 2006;**24**:611-620. DOI: 10.1590/S0100-83582006000400001

[25] Ratnasekera D. Weedy rice: A threat to rice production in Sri Lanka. Journal of the University of Ruhuna. 2015;**3**:2-13. DOI: 10.4038/jur.v3i1.7859

[26] Thurber CS, Hepler PK, Caicedo AL. Timing is everything: Early degradation of abscission layer is associated with increased seed shattering in US weedy rice. BMC Plant Biology. 2011;**11**:14. DOI: 10.1186/1471-2229-11-14

[27] Anuwar Nur Hidayatul SA, Mazlan N, Engku Ahmad KEA, Juraimi AS, Yusop MR. A comparative study of vegetative and reproductive growth of local weedy and Clearfield® rice varieties in Malaysia. Journal of ISSAAS. 2014;**20**:41-51. ISSN: 0859-3132

[28] Burgos NR, Norman RJ, Gealy DR, Black H. Competitive N uptake between rice and weedy rice. Field Crops Research. 2006;**99**:96-105. DOI: 10.1016/j.fcr.2006.03.009

[29] Sales MA, Burgos NR, Shivrain VK, Murphy B, Gbur EE. Morphological and physiological responses of weedy red rice (*Oryza sativa* L.) and cultivated rice (*O. sativa*) to N supply. American Journal of Plant Sciences. 2011;**2**:569-577. DOI: 10.4236/ajps.2011.24068

[30] Ziska LH, McClung A. Differential response of cultivated and weedy (red) rice to recent and projected increases in atmospheric carbon dioxide. Agronomy Journal. 2008;**100**:1259-1263. DOI: 10.2134/agronj2007.0324

[31] Bevilacqua CB, Basu S, Pereira A, Tseng TM, Zimmer PD, Burgos NR. Analysis of stress-responsive gene expression in cultivated and weedy Rice differing in cold stress tolerance. PLoS One. 2015;**10**:e0132100. DOI: 10.1371/journal.pone.0132100

[32] Uddin MK, Dandan HM, Alidin AH. Salinity effects on germination of malaysian rice varieties and weedy rice biotypes. World Academy of Science, Engineering and Technology, International Journal of Bioengineering and Life Sciences. 2015;**2**:724. DOI: 10.12692/ijb/9.3.122-128

[33] Pantone DJ, Baker JB. Weed-crop competition models and response-surface analysis of red rice competition in cultivated rice: A review. Crop Science. 1991;**31**:1105-1110. DOI: 10.2135/cropsci1991.0011183X003100050003x

[34] Ottis BV, Smith KL, Scott RC, Talbert RE. Rice yield and quality as affected by cultivar and red rice (*Oryza sativa*) density. Weed Science. 2005;**53**:499-504. DOI: 10.1614/WS-04-154R

[35] Londo JP, Schaal BA. Origins and population genetics of weedy red rice in the USA. Molecular Ecology. 2007;**16**:4523-4535. DOI: 10.1111/j.1365-294X.2007.03489.x

[36] Kanapeckas KL, Tseng TM, Vigueira CC, Ortiz A, JrBridges WC, Burgos NR, et al. Contrasting patterns of variation in weedy traits and unique crop features in divergent populations of US weedy rice (*Oryza sativa* sp.) in Arkansas and California. Pest Management Science;**2017, 74**:1404-1415. DOI: 10.1002/ps.4820

[37] Burgos NR, Singh V, Tseng TM, Black H, Young ND, Huang Z, et al. The impact of herbicide-resistant rice technology on phenotypic diversity and population structure of United States weedy rice. Plant Physiology. 2014;**114**:242719. DOI: 10.1104/pp.114.242719

[38] Tseng TM. Genetic diversity of seed dormancy and molecular evolution of weedy red rice [PhD dissertation]. University of Arkansas; 2013. Available from: http://scholarworks.uark.edu/etd/595

[39] Ellstrand NC, Heredia SM, Leak-Garcia JA, et al. Crops gone wild: Evolution of weeds and invasives from domesticated ancestors. Evolutionary Applications. 2010;**3**(5-6):494-504. DOI: 10.1111/j.1752-4571.2010.00140.x

[40] De-Wet JMJ, Harlan JR. Weeds and domesticates: Evolution in the man-made habitat. Economic Botany. 1975;**29**:99. DOI: 10.1007/ BF02863309

[41] Cao Q, Lu B-R, Xia H, Rong J, Sala F, Spada A, et al. Genetic diversity and origin of weedy rice (*Oryza sativa f. spontanea*) populations found in North-Eastern China revealed by simple sequence repeat (SSR) markers. Annals of Botany. 2006;**98**:1241-1252. DOI: 10.1093/aob/mcl210

[42] Gealy DR, Agrama HA, Eizenga GC. Exploring genetic and spatial structure of U.S. weedy red rice (*Oryza sativa*) in relation to rice relatives worldwide. Weed Science. 2009;**57**(06):627-643. DOI: 10.1614/WS-09-018.1

[43] Gealy DR. Gene movement between rice (*Oryza sativa*) and weedy rice (*Oryza sativa*): A U.S. temperate rice perspective. In: Gressel J, editor. Crop Ferality and Volunteerism. Boca Raton, FL: CRC Press; 2005. pp. 323-354. DOI: 10.1201/9781420037999.ch20

[44] Pritchard JK, Stephens M, Donnelly P. Inference of population structure using multilocus genotype data. Genetics. 2000;**155**:945-959

[45] Shivrain VK, Burgos NR, Scott RC, Gbur EE Jr, Estorninos LE Jr, McClelland MR. Diversity of weedy red rice (*Oryza sativa* L.) in Arkansas, USA in relation to weed management. Crop Protection. 2010;**29**(7):721-730. DOI: 10.1016/j.cropro.2010.02.010

[46] Chauhan BS, Johnson DE. The role of seed ecology in improving weed management strategies in the tropics. Advances in Agronomy. 2010;**105**: 221-262. DOI: 10.1016/S0065-2113(10)05006-6

[47] Perera UIP, Senanayake SGJN, Ratnasekera WADPR. Morphological diversity of weedy rice accessions

collected in Ampara district. In: Proceedings of International Forestry and Environment Symposium. 2012. p. 15. DOI: 10.31357/fesympo.v15i0. 180.g87

[48] Sudianto E, Neik TX, Tam SM, Chuah TS, Idris AA, Olsen KM, et al. Morphology of Malaysian weedy rice (*Oryza sativa*): Diversity, origin and implications for weed management. Weed Science. 2016;**64**:501-512. DOI: 10.1614/WS-D-15-00168.1

[49] Fogliatto S, Vidotto F, Ferrero A. Morphological characterization of Italian weedy rice (*Oryza sativa*) populations. Weed Research. 2012;**52**:60-69. DOI: 10.1111/j.1365-3180.2011.00890.x

[50] Chen LJ, Lee DS, Song ZP, Suh HS, Lu BR. Gene flow from cultivated rice (*Oryza sativa*) to its weedy and wild relatives. Annals of Botany. 2004;**93**: 67-73. DOI: 10.1093/aob/mch006

[51] Mao-bai L, Hui W, Li-ming C. Evaluation of population structure, genetic diversity and origin of Northeast Asia weedy rice based on simple sequence repeat markers. Rice Science. 2015;**22**:180-188. DOI: 10.1016/j. rsci.2015.02.001

[52] Yu GQ, Bao Y, Shi CH, Dong CQ, Ge S. Genetic diversity and population differentiation of Liaoning weedy rice detected by RAPD and SSR markers. Biochemical Genetics. 2005;**43**:261-270. DOI: 10.1007/s10528-005-5218-3

[53] Gealy DR, Tai TH, Sneller CH. Identification of red rice, rice, and hybrid populations using microsatellite markers. Weed Science. 2002;**50**:333-339. DOI: 10.1614/0043-1745(2002)050[0333,IOR RRA]2.0.CO;2

[54] Shivrain VK, Burgos NR, Agrama HA, Lawton-Rauh A, Lu B, Sales MA, et al. Genetic diversity of weedy red rice (*Oryza sativa*) in Arkansas, USA. Weed Research. 2010;**50**:289-302. DOI: 10.1111/j.1365-3180.2010.00780.x

[55] Reagon M, Thurber CS, Gross BL, Olsen KM, Jia Y, Caicedo AL. Genomic patterns of nucleotide diversity in divergent populations of US weedy rice. BMC Evolutionary Biology. 2010;**10**:180. DOI: 10.1186/1471-2148-10-180

[56] Grimm A, Fogliatto S, Nick P, Ferrero A, Vidotto F. Microsatellite markers reveal multiple origins for Italian weedy rice. Ecology and Evolution. 2013;**3**:4786-4798. DOI: 10.1002/ece3.848

[57] Federici MT, Vaughan D, Norihiko T, Kaga A, Xin WW, Koji D, et al. Analysis of Uruguayan weedy rice genetic diversity using AFLP molecular markers. Electronic Journal of Biotechnology. 2001;**4**:5-6. DOI: 10.2225/vol4-issue3-fulltext-3

[58] Song ZP, Zhu YG, Chen JK. Gene flow from cultivated rice to the wild species *Oryza rufipogon* under experimental field conditions. New Phytologist. 2003;**157**:67-665. DOI: 10.1046/j.1469-8137.2003.00699.x

[59] Gealy DR, Mitten DH, Rutger JN. Gene flow between red rice (*Oryza sativa*) and herbicide-resistant rice (*O. sativa*): Implications for weed management. Weed Technology. 2003;**17**:627-645. DOI: 10.1614/ WT02-100

Section 4

Population Genetics for Conservation Studies

Chapter 4

The Research of Population Genetic Differentiation for Marine Fishes (*Hyporthodus septemfasciatus*) Based on Fluorescent AFLP Markers

Yongshuang Xiao, Zhizhong Xiao, Jing Liu, Daoyuan Ma, Qinghua Liu and Jun Li

Abstract

Hyporthodus septemfasciatus is a commercially important proliferation fish which is distributed in the coastal waters of Japan, Korea, and China. We used the fluorescent AFLP technique to check the genetic differentiations between broodstock and offspring populations. A total of 422 polymorphic bands (70.10%) were detected from the 602 amplified bands. A total of 308 polymorphic loci were checked for broodstock I ($P_{\text{broodstock I}}$ = 55.50%) coupled with 356 and 294 for broodstock II ($P_{\text{broodstock II}}$ = 63.12%) and offspring ($P_{\text{offspring}}$ = 52.88%), respectively. The levels of population genetic diversities for broodstock were higher than those for offspring. Both AMOVA and F_{st} analyses showed that significant genetic differentiation existed among populations, and limited fishery recruitment to the offspring was detected. STRUCTURE and PCoA analyses indicated that two management units existed and most offspring individuals (95.0%) only originated from 44.0% of the individuals of broodstock I, which may have negative effects on sustainable fry production.

Keywords: genetic diversity, population structure, fluorescent AFLP technology, *Hyporthodus septemfasciatus*, sustainable management

1. Introduction

Genetic diversity is one of the most important natural properties for commercially interesting species, because it can influence the species' adaptive capacity to environmental change, and loss of genetic variation is destructive to domestication of cultured stocks [1, 2]. Limited effective population size and the effects of artificial selection on hatchery progeny may lead to population genetic drift, which will cause offspring to differentiate from broodstock [3]. Monitoring population genetic diversity and genetic structure, therefore, has become a key aspect and long-term mission for the success of commercial breeding programs [4].

 IntechOpen

Seven-band grouper, *H. septemfasciatus* (Thunberg, 1793), belongs to the family Serranidae and is distributed in waters of Korea, Japan, and China. It is a sedentary, reef-associated species and lives in shallow water (5–30 m) [4]. *H. septemfasciatus* is a commercially important marine fish with rapid growth and low-temperature tolerance characteristics, which make the species as proliferation fish for cage culture and marine ranching in the coastal waters of Japan, Korea, and China [4–6]. Although the artificial breeding processes for *H. septemfasciatus* have been established, crucial technique problems of artificial breeding with female-fish sex reverse, artificial induction of natural spawning, and treatment of virus diseases for hatched larvae are needed to be solved urgently [4, 5]. Seven-band grouper is a protogynous hermaphrodite fish, which begins life as a female before becoming a male. Until now, almost all of seven-band grouper hatcheries maintain wild-caught sources of *H. septemfasciatus* as broodstock for artificial reproduction [4]. The limited male broodstock (given the extended maturation age) may limit the genetic diversity in breeding programs [3]. The excellent traits for species were always derived from rich genetic variations. In order to avoid the detrimental loss of genetic variation during the artificial propagation process, it is necessary to frequently monitor the genetic diversity and population structure for *H. septemfasciatus*.

Research reports of genetic diversity and population structure between wild and hatchery populations of *H. septemfasciatus* have been carried out based on the microsatellite DNA loci [3, 4]. These genetic studies revealed reduced genetic variability in hatchery populations compared with wild populations, based on microsatellite analyses. Significant population genetic differentiation was also examined among the hatchery population in South Korea [3, 4]. AFLP is a PCR-based, multi-locus fingerprinting technique that can detect genetic variations effectively. It combines the strengths and overcomes the weaknesses of the RFLP and RAPD methods. Until now, AFLP has been proven to be successful in studying population genetic structure and differentiation of plants, animals, and some fish species such as *Carassius auratus*, *Pleuronectes yokohamae*, and *Synechogobius ommaturus*. Until now, research of the population diversity and genetic differentiation between broodstock and offspring from Japan was not reported. In the present research, different fluorescent AFLP markers were used to estimate population genetic variabilities of broodstock and offspring from Japan and Korea. The results will provide a useful genetic basis for future planning of sustainable culture and management of *H. septemfasciatus* in fisheries.

2. Population genetic differentiation for marine fishes based on fluorescent AFLP markers

2.1 Materials and methods

2.1.1 Material information

Sixty-two specimens with two broodstock and one offspring populations were gathered from Korea (broodstock II), Japan (broodstock I), and China (offspring—Rizhao) during May 2014 to September 2014 (**Figure 1**, **Table 1**). We used the *Epinephelus moara* as an outgroup with six individuals sampled from Guangzhou. The taxonomic status of 62 specimens was confirmed based on the measures and segment features, and the fin-clip tissue was collected from each specimen and preserved in 100% ethanol.

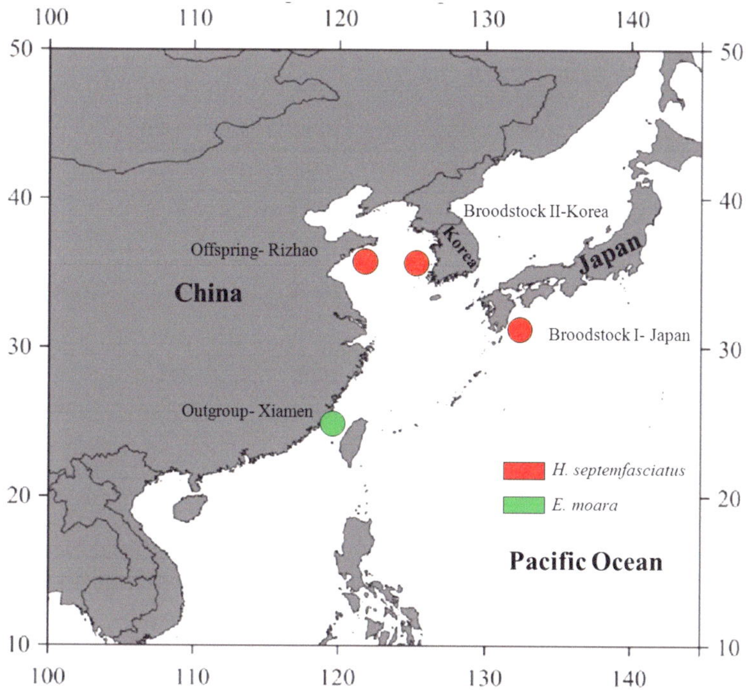

Figure 1.
Sampling location of H. septemfasciatus.

2.1.2 Genomic DNA extraction and AFLP processes

We used a standard phenol-chloroform method to extract the genomic DNA from the fin-clip tissue with proteinase K digestion. The process of AFLP experiment was followed with the procedures developed by Vos et al. [7] and Wang et al. [8]. The genomic DNA with about 100 ng was digested using 1 unit of *Eco*RI and *Mse* I (New England Biolabs Inc., UK) at 37°C for 6 h. We used the ligation system with 1 μL 10× ligation buffer, 5 pmol *Eco*RI adapter (*Eco*RI-1/*Eco*RI-2; **Table 1**), 50 pmol *Mse*I adapter (*Mse*I-1/*Mse*I-2; **Table 1**), and 0.3 unit of T4 DNA ligase (Takara Bio Inc., China) to ligate double-stranded adapters and the restriction fragments together at 20°C overnight. We used TaKaRa Thermal Cycler to conduct the pre-amplification PCR for AFLP with a pair of primers including a single selective nucleotide. The annealing temperature for amplification was 53°C with length of 30 s. Then, the PCR product was diluted tenfold and used as templates for the subsequent selective PCR amplification. We used the FAM fluorescent to label the primer *Eco*RI (FAM-E-AAC, FAM-E-ACA, FAM-E-ACC) (**Table 1**). We used the PCR system with 1 μL pre-amplification product, 1× PCR buffer, 150 μM of each dNTP, 30 ng of each selective primer, and 0.5 unit of *Taq* DNA polymerase to conduct the selective amplifications. The gradient thermocycler with a touchdown cycling procedure of nine cycles of 30 s at 94°C, 30 s at 65°C (−1°C at each cycle), and 30 s at 72°C followed by the cycling procedure of 28 cycles of 30 s at 94°C, 30 s at 56°C, and 1 min at 72°C was used to PCR. The final step was a prolonged extension at 72°C with the length of 7 min. The quality of selective amplification product was checked by electrophoresis in a 4% denaturing polyacrylamide gel (DPG) at 50 W (maximum to 3,000 V) for 2.4 h in ABI Prism 377 DNA Sequencer (Applied Biosystems, USA). Sequences of AFLP adapters and primers are listed in **Table 1**.

Primer pairs	Population	*I*	*He*	*Ne*	*Hw*/*Ht*	G_{st}
FAM-E-AAC/M-CTC	Rizhao	0.190 ± 0.029	0.125 ± 0.020	1.211 ± 0.037	0.200/0.227	0.116
	Japan	0.199 ± 0.030	0.131 ± 0.021	1.223 ± 0.038		
	Korea	0.266 ± 0.031	0.176 ± 0.022	1.297 ± 0.040		
	Average	0.218 ± 0.017	0.144 ± 0.012	1.244 ± 0.022		
	E. moara	0.152 ± 0.027	0.098 ± 0.018	1.162 ± 0.034		
FAM-E-AAC/M-CTG	Rizhao	0.234 ± 0.027	0.153 ± 0.018	1.249 ± 0.032	0.229/0.256	0.107
	Japan	0.232 ± 0.027	0.153 ± 0.019	1.260 ± 0.036		
	Korea	0.272 ± 0.027	0.177 ± 0.019	1.290 ± 0.034		
	Average	0.246 ± 0.016	0.161 ± 0.011	1.266 ± 0.019		
	E. moara	0.195 ± 0.027	0.130 ± 0.019	1.225 ± 0.036		
FAM-E-ACA/M-CAT	Rizhao	0.196 ± 0.024	0.129 ± 0.017	1.214 ± 0.030	0.199/0.249	0.197
	Japan	0.242 ± 0.025	0.159 ± 0.017	1.265 ± 0.032		
	Korea	0.237 ± 0.025	0.155 ± 0.017	1.260 ± 0.032		
	Average	0.225 ± 0.014	0.148 ± 0.010	1.246 ± 0.018		
	E. moara	0.157 ± 0.023	0.104 ± 0.016	1.176 ± 0.029		
FAM-E-ACA/M-CTT	Rizhao	0.254 ± 0.024	0.168 ± 0.017	1.284 ± 0.030	0.234/0.266	0.119
	Japan	0.227 ± 0.023	0.148 ± 0.016	1.250 ± 0.030		
	Korea	0.306 ± 0.024	0.201 ± 0.017	1.338 ± 0.031		
	Average	0.262 ± 0.014	0.173 ± 0.010	1.291 ± 0.018		
	E. moara	0.150 ± 0.022	0.102 ± 0.015	1.180 ± 0.029		
FAM-E-ACC/M-ACT	Rizhao	0.298 ± 0.022	0.199 ± 0.016	1.343 ± 0.029	0.257/0.285	0.099
	Japan	0.287 ± 0.022	0.191 ± 0.016	1.328 ± 0.029		
	Korea	0.305 ± 0.021	0.201 ± 0.015	1.340 ± 0.029		
	Average	0.297 ± 0.013	0.197 ± 0.009	1.337 ± 0.017		
	E. moara	0.234 ± 0.022	0.157 ± 0.016	1.274 ± 0.029		
Total	Rizhao	0.243 ± 0.011	0.161 ± 0.008	1.271 ± 0.014	0.229/0.261	0.124
	Japan	0.244 ± 0.011	0.161 ± 0.008	1.272 ± 0.015		
	Korea	0.281 ± 0.011	0.185 ± 0.008	1.310 ± 0.015		
	Average	0.256 ± 0.007	0.169 ± 0.005	1.284 ± 0.008		
	E. moara	0.182 ± 0.011	0.121 ± 0.008	1.210 ± 0.014		

I, Shannon diversity index; He, expected heterozygosity; Ne, no. of effective alleles; Hw, gene diversity within populations; Ht, population genetic structure.

Table 1.
Parameters of genetic diversity for three populations of H. septemfasciatus.

Similarity indices were calculated using the formula S = 2Nab/(Na + Nb), where Na and Nb were the number of bands in individuals a and b, respectively, and Nab was the number of sharing bands. Genetic distances between individuals were computed using the formula D = −ln S. Genetic relationship among populations was constructed based on unweighted pair-group method analysis (UPGMA) by TFPGA [9].

2.2 Data analysis

2.2.1 AFLP data analysis

We used the ABI 3730xl Genetic Analyzer (Applied Biosystems) to check the PCR products, which were genotyped by using the internal size standard LIZ 500 (Applied Biosystems) and scored using the GeneScan3.1 software (Applied Biosystems) in Shanghai Personal Biotechnology Co., Ltd.

2.2.2 Genetic variability parameter analyses

The fragment size with length ranging from 70 to 1000 bp was used for further analyses. Firstly, the clear and unambiguous AFLP bands were scored with 1 or 0, and then we transformed the bands into 0/1 binary matrix. The genetic variability parameters with polymorphic bands, effective number of alleles per loci (*Ne*), expected heterozygosity (*H*), Shannon's information index (*I*), and Nei's genetic distances were calculated by GenALEx 6.501 [10]. The parameters of genetic structure (*Ht*) among populations were also evaluated by AFLP-SURV [11].

Genetic differentiation between population pairs was evaluated by fixation indices F_{st} and Nei's genetic distance using Arlequin [12] and GenALEx 6.501 [10] software. When multiple comparisons were performed, *P* values were adjusted using the sequential Bonferroni procedure. Analysis of molecular variance (AMOVA) [13] was employed to further examine hierarchical population structure as well as the geographical pattern of population subdivision [13]. We used the software STRUCTURE version 2.3.3 with a Bayesian model to evaluate genetic structures of the *H. septemfasciatus* populations [14]. The admixture model and independent allelic frequencies were used to analyze the data set and the length of the burn-in period and a number of MCMC reps after burn-in were set to 25,000 and 100,000, respectively. These steps were used to determine the ancestry value, which estimated the proportion of an individual's genome that originated from a given genetic group. The algorithm was run 10 times for each K value, from 1 to 4.

2.3 Results

2.3.1 Polymorphic information of different AFLP primers

To remove false-positive bands, a total of 602 clear and unambiguous bands were detected from two broodstock and one offspring populations by using five-pair selective primers. A total of 422 polymorphic bands (70.10%) were detected from the 602 amplified bands (**Table 1**). The average bands of polymorphic sites for five-pair primers were 84.4, which were ranged from 52 to 129 (**Table 1**). The maximum of polymorphic bands was detected in the FAM-E-ACC/M-ACT primer pair (129 bands), and the minimum of polymorphic bands was found in the FAM-E-AAC/M-CTC primer pair (52 bands). Three hundred and eight polymorphic loci were checked for broodstock I ($P_{\text{broodstock I}}$ = 55.50%) coupled with 356 and 294 for broodstock II ($P_{\text{broodstock II}}$ = 63.12%) and offspring ($P_{\text{offspring}}$ = 52.88%), respectively. Different patterns of polymorphic sites were detected between broodstock and offspring populations of *H. septemfasciatus* from the same primer pair. Two hundred and eighty-five bands were found from the individuals of *E. moara*, 74.74% of which (213) were polymorphic (**Table 1**). Special bands were also detected based on the five-pair selective primers, which ranged from 1 to 11 for broodstock I (Japan, n = 1), broodstock II (Korea, n = 11), and offspring (n = 8) populations (**Table 1**, **Figure 2**). The number of special bands was 317 for *E. moara* compared with *H. septemfasciatus*.

2.3.2 Genetic variability of *H. septemfasciatus*

The average values of *Ne* for broodstock I (Japan), broodstock II (Korea), and offspring were 1.272 ± 0.015, 1.310 ± 0.015, and 1.271 ± 0.014, respectively. The effective alleles of broodstock II (Korea) were higher than that of broodstock I (Japan). And the average value of *Ne* for both broodstock and offspring populations was 1.284 ± 0.008. The average value of expected heterozygosity for broodstock II population was higher than those of broodstock I (*He* = 0.161 ± 0.008) and offspring (*He* = 0.161 ± 0.008) populations. The homogeneous trend was also detected from the parameter of Shannon diversity index (*I*) in broodstock ($I_{\text{broodstock II}}$ = 0.281 ± 0.011 and $I_{\text{broodstock I}}$ = 0.244 ± 0.011) and offspring ($I_{\text{offspring}}$ = 0.243 ± 0.011) populations. The total *He* and *I* for the three populations of *H. septemfasciatus* were 0.169 ± 0.005 and 0.256 ± 0.007, respectively. The parameter of genetic diversity within population (*Hw*) ranged from 0.199 to 0.257, and the average value of *Hw* was 0.229 for the three populations (**Table 1**). According to the results of *Ne*, *He*, and *I* parameters, although different primer pairs showed different levels of genetic diversity, the broodstock II showed the highest level of genetic diversity among the three populations (**Table 1**).

Though the five primer pairs showed different genetic differentiations among populations, the values of genetic structure (*Ht*) parameter ranged from 0.227 to 0.285, which showed significant genetic structure existed among populations

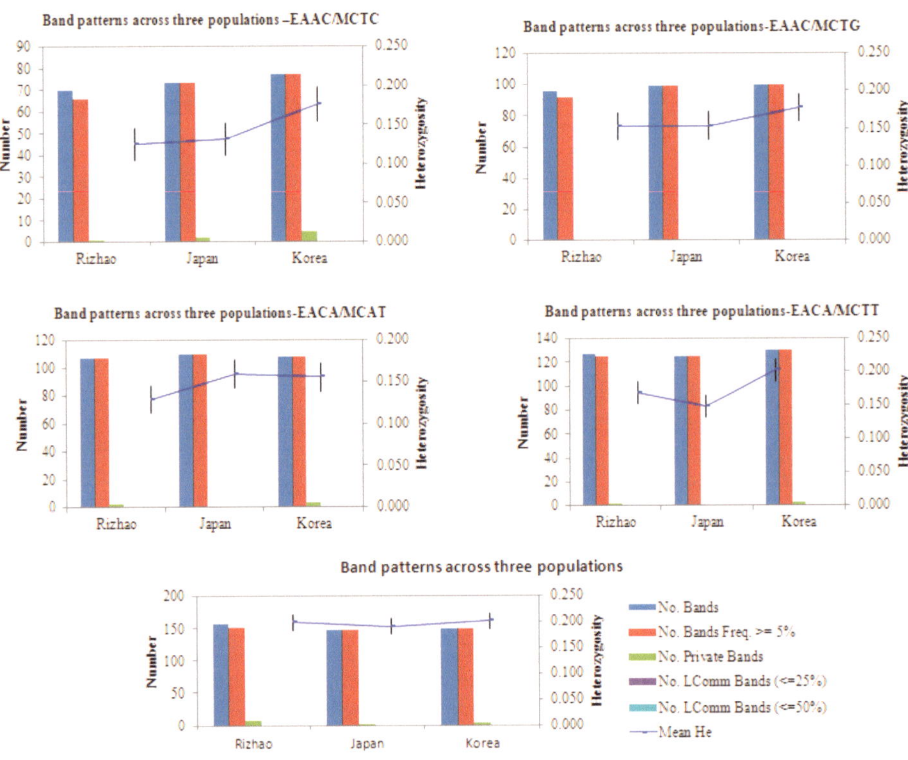

Figure 2.
Number of bands based on different AFLP primers for H. septemfasciatus.

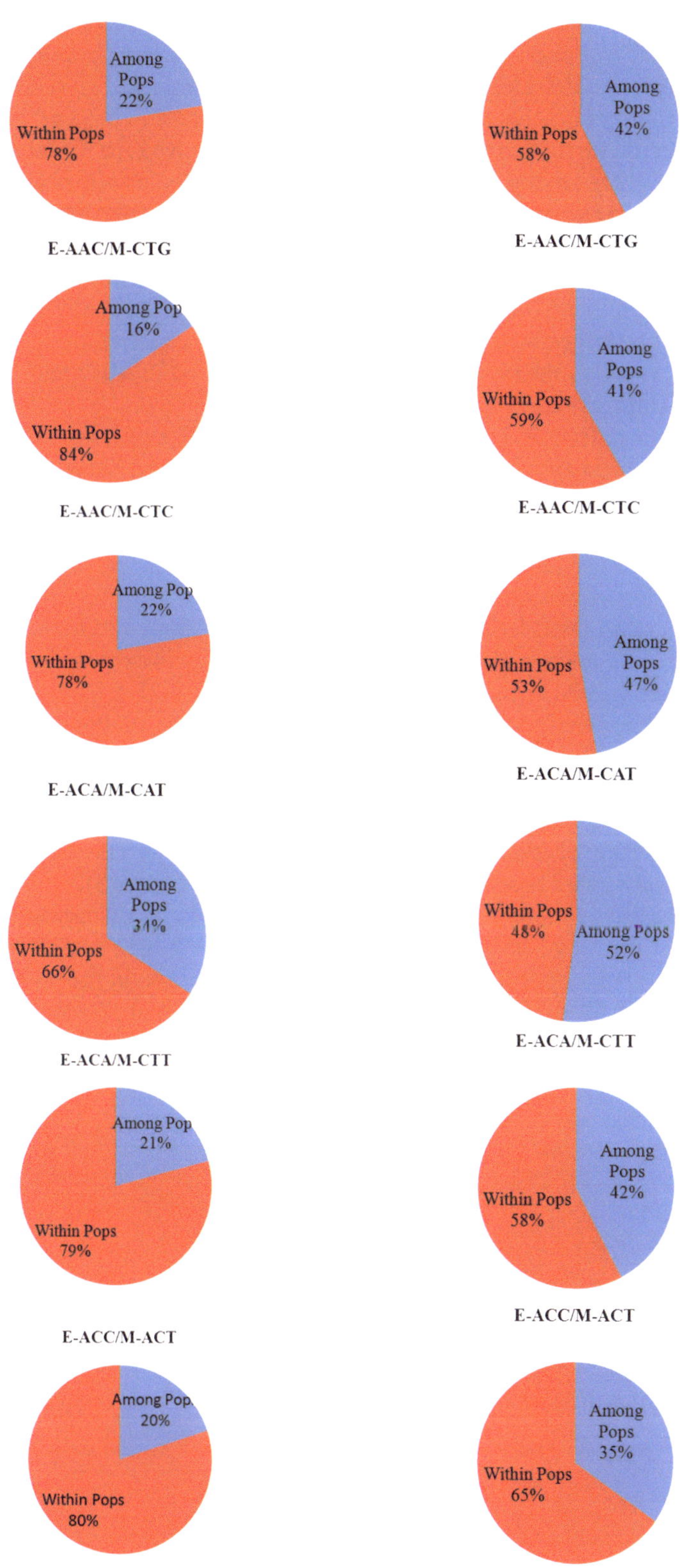

Figure 3.
AMOVAs based on different AFLP primers for H. septemfasciatus.

(**Table 1**). The AMOVA showed that 77.63% of variation was derived within populations and 22.37% of genetic variation happened among populations. The genetic variations were further estimated by each of the five primer pairs, which indicated more than 15.83% genetic variation originated from the variation among populations. In addition to the AMOVA and *Ht*, the values of genetic differentiation ranged from 0.099 to 0.197 based on the G_{st} parameters (**Figure 3**). The genetic structure was also detected by the pairwise F_{st} analysis, which showed the F_{st} values ranging from 0.169 to 0.292 among broodstock and offspring populations (**Figure 4**). And the largest value was detected between Korea and offspring (F_{st} = 0.292, P < 0.01) populations, whereas the lowest value was found between Japan and Korea (F_{st} = 0.169, P < 0.01) populations. The Nei's genetic distances among populations were ranged from 0.048 to 0.083. The result was similar with the pairwise F_{st} analysis, and the largest value was found between Korea and offspring (D = 0.083) populations, whereas the lowest value was checked between Japan and Korea (D = 0.048) populations (**Figure 5**).

We used the software of STRUCTURE to estimate the ancestor composition based on the coalescent theory. Three clusters were checked between broodstock and offspring populations based on a clear maximum for ΔK at K = 3 calculated by the MCMC method (**Figures 6** and 7). Cluster 1 was mainly composed of offspring (F = 95.0%) and broodstock I (Japan, F = 44.0%) populations, and the contribution of broodstock II (Korea) to the offspring was only 9.1%. Cluster 3 was mainly originated from the broodstock I (F = 55.9%) and broodstock II (F = 90.3%), and the contribution of them to the offspring was only 4.9%. Cluster 2 was occupied by all the individuals of *E. moara* (F = 98.1%). Three groups of the specimens were also verified by principal coordinates analysis (PCoA), which showed the individuals of offspring population being derived from the broodstock I and broodstock II, respectively. The individuals of *E. moara* formed the independent group (**Figure 8**).

The relationship of individuals was further illustrated by a dendrogram using the UPGMA algorithm based on Nei's genetic distance (**Figure 5**). Significant genealogical structure was detected in *H. septemfasciatus*. The dendrogram showed that three significant genealogical branches (Clade A, Clade B, and outgroup) corresponding to sampling localities of Japan and Korea existed in the species, respectively (**Figure 9**). Clade A was composed of Korea population. Most individuals of

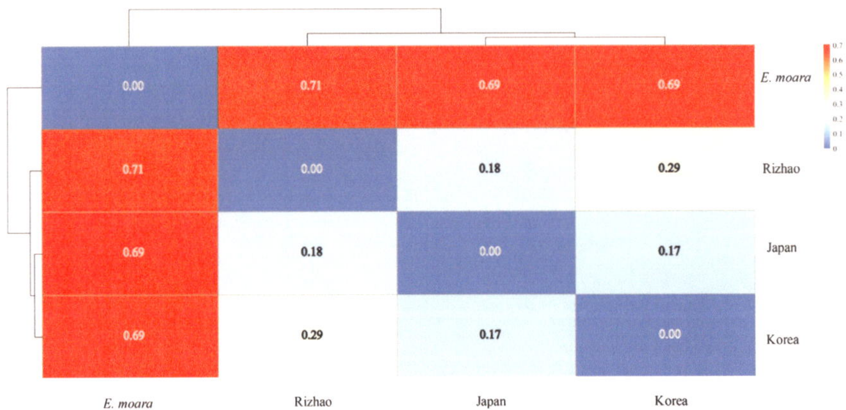

Figure 4.
Pairwise F_{st} among populations of H. septemfasciatus. All of the values were significant (p < 0.01).

DOI: http://dx.doi.org/10.5772/intechopen.81796

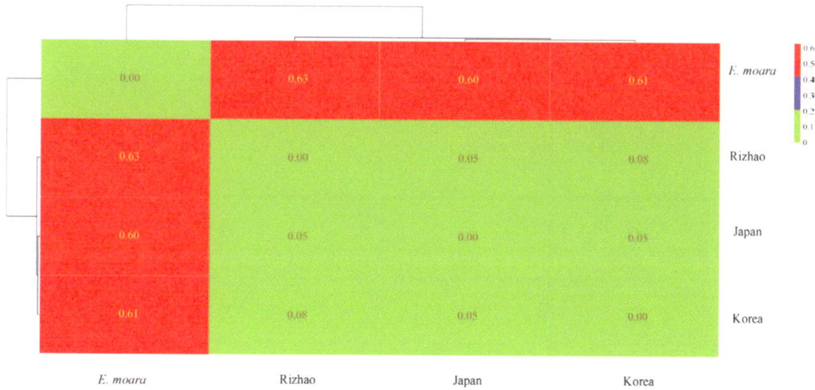

Figure 5.
Nei's genetic distance among populations of H. septemfasciatus.

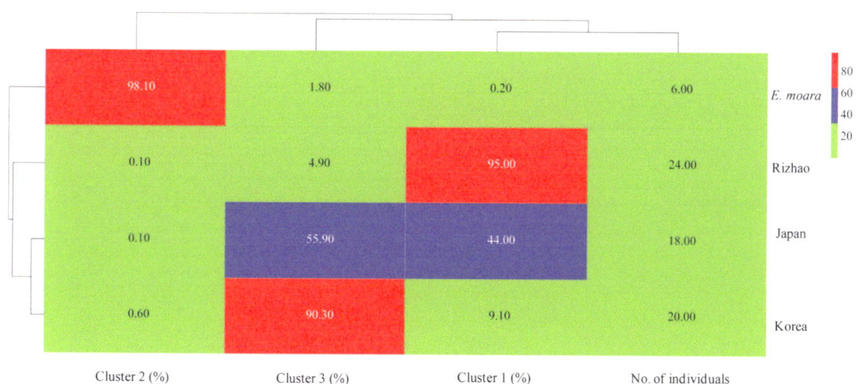

Figure 6.
The distribution of individuals of three populations in two genetic groups inferred by STRUCTURE.

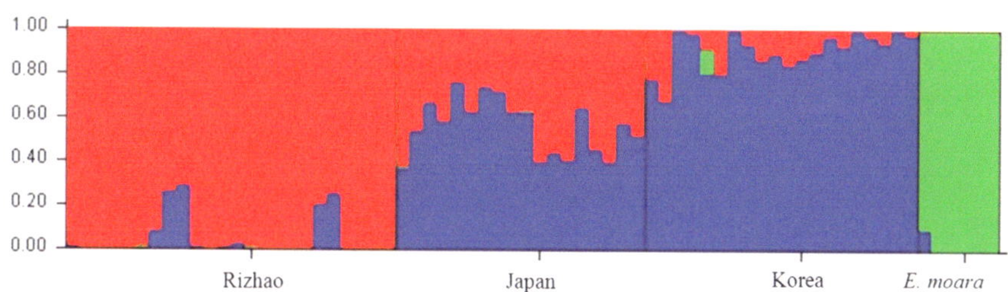

Figure 7.
Clustering of three populations for H. septemfasciatus. Each individual is shown as a vertical line divided into segments representing the estimated membership proportion in the three ancestral genetic clusters inferred from STRUCTURE.

Japan population and whole individuals of Rizhao population formed Clade B. The relationship among populations was also carried out based on Nei's genetic distance by TFPGA, and near relationship between Japan and Rizhao populations was checked.

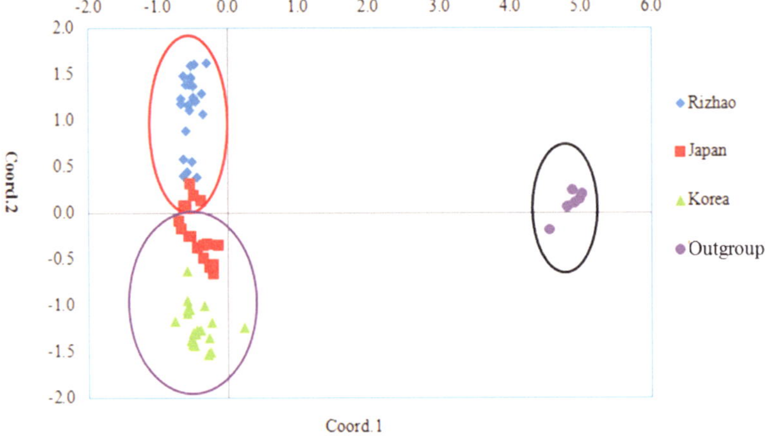

Figure 8.
Principal coordinates analysis (PCoA) of three populations of H. septemfasciatus.

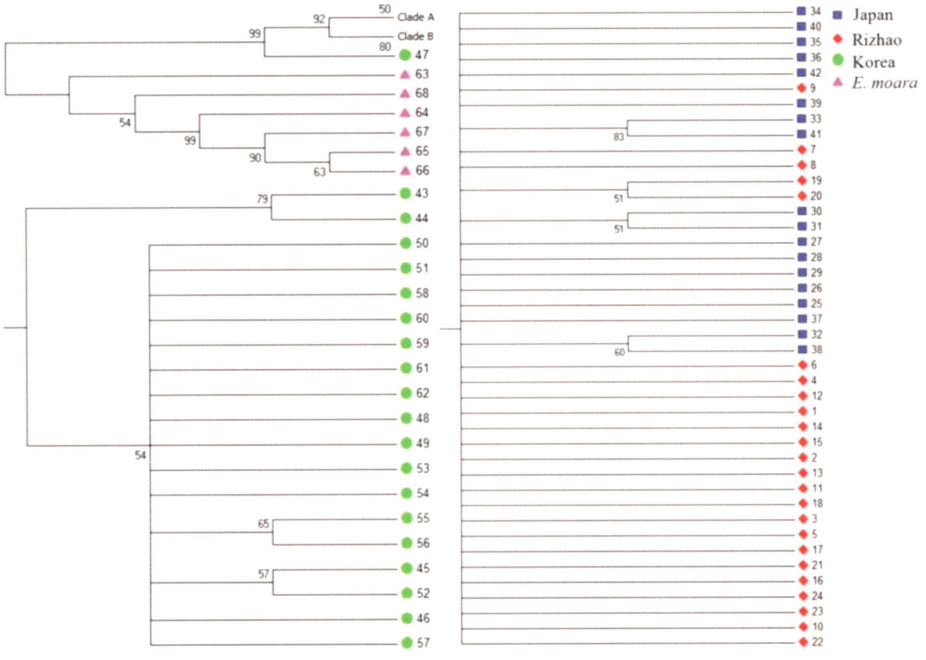

Figure 9.
UPGMA tree of individuals of H. septemfasciatus based on Nei's genetic distance.

3. Conclusions

In this study, significant genetic differentiations were checked among the broodstock and offspring populations of *H. septemfasciatus* by using F_{st}, AMOVA, and STRUCTURE analyses. The broodstock I population from Japan was a significant divergent from the broodstock II population from Korea. The contribution of broodstock I (Japan, F = 44.0%) to the offspring population reached up to 95.0%; on the contrary, 55.9% of broodstock I individuals and 90.3% of broodstock II individuals only have contributed 4.9% of individuals to the offspring population.

According to the STRUCTURE, PCoA, and UPGMA algorithm, two management units were checked from the broodstock and offspring populations based on the five fluorescent AFLP primer pairs. The differentiation among populations was not only originated from the genetic variabilities between broodstock I population (Japan) and broodstock II populations (Korea) but also originated from the low number of founding individuals in the hatcheries, especially for the broodstock II (Korea). The passive founder effect could lead to serious genetic drift and significant genetic differentiation, which has been well documented in other fish species [15].

High level of polymorphic sites (70.10%) was detected for *H. septemfasciatus* based on the fluorescent AFLP technique, which was higher than those of other fishes using general AFLP technique (18.6–55.8%) [16, 17]. We checked significant degradation of genetic diversity in the two broodstock and one offspring populations of *H. septemfasciatus* (P = 70.10%, I = 0.256, H_e = 0.169, N_e = 1.284) compared with wild populations (P = 98.73%, I = 0.288, H_e = 0.189, N_e = 1.319) of other rock reef fish species using fluorescent AFLP with similar primer pairs [18]. The parameters of genetic diversity in the wild-caught broodstock II population (I = 0.281, H_e = 0.185, N_e = 1.310) from Korea was higher than that of wild-caught broodstock I population (I = 0.244, H_e = 0.161, N_e = 1.272) from Japan. The level of genetic diversity of offspring population was similar with that of broodstock I population from Japan.

The genetic variability is one of the most crucial foundations for the conservation of marine species from long-time objective. Although significant degradation of genetic variations has been previously reported between broodstock and offspring in other marine fishes, no significant reduction of genetic diversity was checked between broodstock I (Japan, I = 0.244, H_e = 0.161, N_e = 1.272) and offspring (I = 0.243, H_e = 0.161, N_e = 1.271) populations in this study [3, 4, 19]. High levels of genetic diversity in wild populations of fish can be related to large effective population size, environmental heterogeneity, life history traits, and genetic divergence [18]. The value of heterozygosity derived from significant geographic difference for *Mugil cephalus* in coastal waters of China was higher than that in Florida based on AFLP analysis [20, 21]. The offspring population of *H. septemfasciatus* may have experienced passive founder effect derived from small population size of broodstock and protogynous hermaphrodite characteristics for grouper fish. Significant reduction of genetic diversity for offspring population may occur compared with broodstock population. On the contrary, the offspring of *H. septemfasciatus* harbored a high level of genetic variability compared with broodstock I population in the present study. Therefore, we believed that significant heterozygosity might exist in the offspring to maintain the high level of genetic diversity.

Significant genetic differentiations were detected between broodstock I population from Japan and broodstock II population from Korea for *H. septemfasciatus* based on AMOVA, F_{st}, STRUCTURE, PCoA, and UPGMA tree analyses. All the results showed that the achieved hatchery progeny of *H. septemfasciatus* might be a composite population originated from broodstock I and broodstock II populations. It was confirmed that the offspring of *H. septemfasciatus* was a composite population, and 95.0% of offspring individuals was derived from 44.0% of broodstock I individuals and 9.1% of broodstock II individuals. The left individuals of offspring (5.0%) were originated from 55.9% of broodstock I individuals and 90.3% of broodstock II individuals. Limited effective population size of the broodstock was always responsible for the pattern of genetic differentiation [3, 4]. Hence, genetic drift has probably played an important role in causing offspring to differentiate from broodstock [4]. In fact, no significant reduction of genetic diversity was checked in the offspring originated from limited population size of broodstock. The offspring of *H. septemfasciatus* was a composite population, which supported the finding for *H. septemfasciatus* with a high level of genetic diversity compared with broodstock I. The present results indicated that broodstock with different genetic backgrounds could make contributions to the maintenance of genetic diversity for compounded offspring. The results of the present study also supported the suggestion that the effective broodstock management procedure be carried out to maintain the genetic diversity of hatchery stocks. It was also reported that added effective population size of broodstock with genetic differentiation backgrounds might be responsible for the reproductive success of grouper [22]. In relation to the management of hatcheries, the geographic sources of different broodstock should be labeled to avoid inbreeding [3, 4]. Hence, continued genetic monitoring of broodstock is necessary for hatchery progeny [3, 4].

Understanding of population genetic diversity and genetic structure has become a key aspect and long-standing issue in speciation and biological conservation. Uncovering the situation of marine population genetic diversity and gene flow is critical for the decision about sustainable exploitation. Evaluating population genetic diversity and structure also can be a vital tool for managing and maintaining a productive fishery [23]. Severe population size declines can also result in the loss of genetic diversity [24]. These results also indicate that genetic drift has led to negative effects on the reproductive capacity of the stock, which may have resulted in significant genetic differentiation between broodstock and offspring populations. The present study of *H. septemfasciatus* indicated at least two management units existed in the wild populations from Japan and Korea, which has supported crucial genetic information to ensure the success of ongoing breeding and stock enhancement programs. Thus, the monitor and management with fixed frequency to hatchery populations will be necessary to ensure the success of artificial seed production [3, 4]. Our data provide a useful genetic basis for future planning of sustainable culture and management of *H. septemfasciatus* in fisheries.

Acknowledgements

This study was supported by a grant from the National Natural Science Foundation of China (No. 41506170, No. 31672672, and No. 31872195), Shandong Province Key Research and Invention Program (2017GHY15102, 2017GHY15106), Qingdao Source Innovation Program (17-1-1-57-jch), Marine Fishery Institute of Zhejiang Province, Key Laboratory of Mariculture and Enhancement of Zhejiang Province (2016KF002), Qingdao National Laboratory for Marine Science and Technology (2015ASKJ02, 2015ASKJ02-03-03), and STS project (KFZD-SW-106, ZSSD-019).

Conflict of interest

The authors declare that they have no competing interests.

Author details

Yongshuang Xiao[1,2,3*†], Zhizhong Xiao[1,2,3†], Jing Liu[1,2,3*], Daoyuan Ma[1,2,3], Qinghua Liu[1,2,3] and Jun Li[1,2,3*]

1 Institute of Oceanology, Chinese Academy of Sciences, Qingdao, China

2 Laboratory for Marine Biology and Biotechnology, Qingdao National Laboratory for Marine Science and Technology, Qingdao, China

3 Center for Ocean Mega-Science, Chinese Academy of Sciences, Qingdao, China

*Address all correspondence to: dahaishuang1982@163.com, jliu@qdio.ac.cn and junli@qdio.ac.cn

† These authors equally contributed to this work.

References

[1] Derek S, Brook BW, Richard F. Most species are not driven to extinction before genetic factors impact them. Proceedings of the National Academy of Sciences of the United States of America. 2004;**101**:15261-15264. DOI: 10.1073/pnas.0403809101

[2] Marja-Liisa K, Riho G, Jarmo K. Wild Estonian and Russian sea trout (*Salmo trutta*) in Finnish coastal sea trout catches: Results of genetic mixed-stock analysis. Hereditas. 2015;**151**:177-195. DOI: 10.1111/hrd2.00070

[3] Hye-Suck A, Jae-Kwon C, Kyong-Min K, Maeng-Hyun S, Jung-Youn P, Jeong-In M, et al. Genetic characterization of four hatchery populations of the seven-band grouper (*Epinephelus septemfasciatus*) using microsatellite markers. Biochemical Systematics and Ecology. 2014;**57**:297-304. DOI: 10.1016/j.bse.2014.08.018

[4] Hye-Suck A, Jae-Kwon C, Kyong-Min K, Maeng-Hyun S, Jung-Youn P, Jeong-In M, et al. Genetic differences between brood stock and offspring of seven-band grouper in a hatchery. Genes & Genomics. 2014;**36**:661-669. DOI: 10.1007/s13258-014-0213-x

[5] Xinfu L, Zhimeng Z, Zhen M, Jilin L, Zhi Y. Progress of artificial breeding technique for seven-band grouper *Epinephelus septemfasciatus*. Journal of Fishery Sciences of China. 2010;**17**:1128-1136. DOI: 1005-8737-(2010)05-1128-09

[6] Ivanchong CK, Ken-ichi Y, Masaharu T, Yasushi T, Hiromi O. Cryopreservation of sperm from seven-band grouper, *Epinephelus septemfasciatus*. Cryobiology. 2010;**61**:263-267. DOI: 10.1016/j.cryobiol.2010.09.003

[7] Pieter V, Rene H, Marjo B, Martin R, Theo NDL, Miranda H, et al. AFLP: A new technique for DNA fingerprinting. Nucleic Acids Research. 1995;**23**:4407-4414. DOI: 10.1093/nar/23.21.4407

[8] Zhiyong W, Yilei W, Limin L, Shuzhen Q, Okamoto N. Genetic polymorphisms in wild and cultured large yellow croaker *Pseudosciaena crocea* using AFLP fingerprinting. Journal of Fishery Sciences of China. 2002;**9**:198-202. DOI: 1005-8737(2002)03-0198-05

[9] Marker PM. Tools for Population Genetic Analyses (TFPGA). A Windows program for the analysis of allozyme and molecular population genetic data version 1.3 [thesis]. Department of Biological Sciences, Northern Arizona University; 1997

[10] Rod P, Peter ES. GENALEX 6.5: Genetic analysis in Excel. Population genetic software for teaching and research—An update. Bioinformatics. 2005;**28**:2537-2539. DOI: 10.1111/j.1471-8286.2005.01155.x

[11] Vekemans X, Beauwens T, Lemaire M, Roldan-Ruiz I. Data from amplified fragment length polymorphism (AFLP) markers show indication of size homoplasy and of a relationship between degree of homoplasy and fragment size. Molecular Ecology. 2002;**11**:139-151. DOI: 10.1046/j.0962-1083.2001.01415.x

[12] Laruent E, Heidi ELL. Arlequin suite ver 3.5: A new series of programs to perform population genetics analyses under Linux and Windows. Molecular Ecology Resources. 2010;**10**:564-567. DOI: 10.1111/j.1755-0998.2010.02847.x

[13] Laurent E, Peter ES, Joseph MQ. Analysis of molecular variance inferred from metric distances among DNA haplotypes: Application to human mitochondrial DNA restriction data.

Genetics. 1992;**131**:2479-2491. PubMed: 1644282

[14] Jonathan KP, Matthew S, Peter D. Inference of population structure using multilocus genotype data. Genetics. 2000;**155**:945-959. PubMed: 10835412

[15] Masashi S, Motoyuki H, Nobuhiko T. Loss of microsatellite and mitochondrial DNA variation in hatchery strains of Japanese flounder *Paralichthys olivaceus*. Aquaculture. 2002;**213**:101-122. DOI: 10.1016/S0044-8486(01)00885-7

[16] Sanlei L, Dongdong X, Lou B, Weiding W, Jian X, Guomin M, et al. The genetic diversity of wild and hatchery-released *Oplegnathus fasciatus* from inshore water of Zhoushan revealed by AFLP. Marine Sciences. 2012;**36**:21-27. DOI: 1000-3096(2012)08-0021-07

[17] Biqian L, Wenqi D, Yajun W, Shihua Z, Wangxing W. Identification of germplasm in *Pseudosciaena crocea* Tai-Chu race by AFLP. Acta Hydrobiologica Sinica. 2005;**29**:413-416. DOI: 1000-3207(2005)04-0413-04

[18] Yongshuang X, Jun L, Guijing R, Daoyuan M, Yanfeng W, Zhizhong X, et al. Pronounced population genetic differentiation in the rock bream *Oplegnathus fasciatus* inferred from mitochondrial DNA sequences. Mitochondrial DNA. 2016;**27**:2045-2052. DOI: 10.3109/19401736.2014.982553

[19] Anne R, Nicholas GE, Peter MG, Catherine C, Richard P, Robert DW. Genetic differentiation between Tasmanian cultured Atlantic salmon (*Salmo salar* L.) and their ancestral Canadian population: Comparison of microsatellite DNA and allozyme and mitochondrial DNA variation. Aquaculture. 1999;**173**:459-469. DOI: 10.1016/S0044-8486(98)00476-1

[20] Donald EC, Behzad MC. Allozyme variation and population structure of striped mullet (*Mugil cephalus*) in Florida. Copeia. 1991;**1991**:485-492. DOI: 10.2307/1446596

[21] Jiangyong L, Zhaorong L, Junbin Z, Tingbao Y. Population genetic structure of striped mullet, *Mugil cephalus*, along the coast of China, inferred by AFLP fingerprinting. Biochemical Systematics and Ecology. 2009;**37**:266-274. DOI: 10.1016/j.bse.2009.04.010

[22] Amos W, Wilmer JW, Fullard K, Burg TM, Croxall JP, Bloch D, et al. The influence of parental relatedness on reproductive success. Proceedings of the Royal Society of London B. 2001;**268**:2021-2027. DOI: 10.1098/rspb.2001.1751

[23] Lisa WS, James ES, Jeffrey JP. Genetic variation in highly exploited spiny lobster *Panulirus marginatus* populations from the Hawaiian archipelago. Fishery Bulletin. 1990;**88**:713-718

[24] Travis CG, Wolfgang S, Michael JB. Effects of a population bottleneck on whooping crane mitochondrial DNA variation. Conservation Biology. 2001;**13**:1097-1107. DOI: 10.1046/j.1523-1739.1999.97527.x